Practical Manual of Echocardiography in the Urgent Setting

To:

– Dr Balendu Vasavada, whose knowledge and dedication to echocardiography has been the basis of this textbook. Many of the images in this book are a direct result of his leadership at the echocardiography laboratory of Long Island College Hospital.

– Dr Steven Bergmann, who served as a great mentor throughout my training and clinical practice. His tremendous assistance and dedication to cardiology have made my career possible.

– Dr Cesare Saponieri, who is responsible for all I know about the practice of clinical cardiology. His pursuit of providing great care to patients is truly an inspiration.

– Of course, Dr Mario Garcia for spending countless hours going through all the text, figures, and tables in this book. Without him, this book would not be possible.

– All of my cardiology colleagues who made this book a reality.

Thank you.

Practical Manual of Echocardiography in the Urgent Setting

EDITED BY

Vladimir Fridman, MD

Cardiovascular Diseases
Brooklyn, NY, USA

Mario J. Garcia, MD

Professor, Department of Medicine (Cardiology)
Professor, Department of Radiology
Chief, Division of Cardiology
Co-Director, Montefiore Einstein Center for Heart and Vascular Care
New York, NY, USA

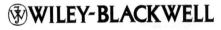

A John Wiley & Sons, Ltd., Publication

Contents

Contributors

Luis Aybar, MD
Cardiovascular Diseases
Beth Israel Medical Center
New York, NY, USA

Salim Baghdadi, MD
Department of Cardiology
Long Island College Hospital
New York, NY, USA

Chirag R. Barbhaiya, MD
Cardiology Fellow
Beth Israel Medical Center
New York, NY, USA

Dimitry Bosoy, MD
Clinical Teaching Attending
Department of Emergency Medicine
Maimonides Medical Center
Brooklyn, NY, USA

Muhammad M. Chaudhry, MD
Cardiology Fellow
Beth Israel Medical Center
New York, NY, USA

Sandeep Dhillon, MD, FACC
Cardiovascular Diseases
Beth Israel Medical Center
New York, NY, USA

Ravi Diwan, MD
Beth Israel Medical Center
New York, NY, USA

Dayana Eslava, MD
St Luke's Roosevelt Hospital
Columbia University College of Physicians and Surgeons
New York, NY, USA

Dennis Finkielstein, MD, FACC, FASE
Director, Ambulatory Cardiology
Program Director, Cardiovascular Diseases Fellowship
Beth Israel Medical Center, New York, NY, USA
Assistant Professor of Medicine
Albert Einstein College of Medicine
New York, NY, USA

Karthik Gujja, MD, MPH
Division of Cardiology
Department of Internal Medicine
Long Island College Hospital
New York, NY, USA

Erika R. Gehrie, MD, FACC
Medical Director, Echocardiography
Preferred Health Partners,
Brooklyn, NY, USA

Yili Huang, DO, FACC
Beth Israel Medical Center
New York, NY, USA

Moinakhtar Lala, MD
Fellow in Cardiovascular Diseases
Cardiovascular Diseases
Beth Israel Medical Center
New York, NY, USA

Michael J. Levine, MD
Cardiovascular Diseases
NYU Langone Medical Center
New York, NY, USA

Vinay Manoranjan Pai, MBBS, MD
Fellow, Cardiovascular Medicine
Beth Israel Medical Center and Long Island College Hospital
New York, NY, USA

Deepika Misra, MBBS, FACC
Beth Israel Medical Center
New York, NY, USA

Sheila Gupta Nadiminti, MD
Department of Cardiology
Beth Israel Medical Center
New York, NY, USA

Hejmadi Prabhu, MD
Cardiovascular Diseases
Wyckoff Heights Medical Center
Brooklyn, NY, USA

Cesare Saponieri, MD, FACC
Electrophysiology and Cardiovascular Diseases
Brooklyn, NY, USA

Jagdeep Singh, MBBS
Cardiovascular Diseases
Beth Israel Medical Center
New York, NY, USA

Padmakshi Singh, MD
Fellow in Cardiovascular Diseases
Cardiovascular Diseases
SUNY Downstate Medical Center
Brooklyn, NY, USA

Sapan Talati, MD
Fellow in Cardiovascular Diseases
SUNY Downstate Medical Center
Brooklyn, NY, USA

Furqan H. Tejani, MD, FACC, FSCCT
Associate Professor of Medicine
Director, Advanced Cardiovascular Imaging
Director, Nuclear Cardiology and Electrocardiography Laboratories
State University of New York
Downstate Medical Center
University Hospital of Brooklyn at Long Island College Hospital
Brooklyn, NY, USA

Alexander Tsukerman, MD, FACEP
Attending, Emergency Medicine
Partner, Emergency Medical Associates
Staten Island, New York, NY, USA

Balendu C. Vasavada, MD, FACC
Director of Echocardiography and Chief of Cardiology Service
University Hospital of Brooklyn at Long Island College Hospital
SUNY Downstate Medical Center
New York, NY, USA

Mariusz W. Wysoczanski, MD
Fellow, Cardiovascular Diseases
Beth Israel Medical Center
Albert Einstein College of Medicine
New York, NY, USA

Preface

There will be times when you will need to read a comprehensive echocardiography textbook. However, there will be also times when you will need to access quick reference information to help you manage a crashing patient in an urgent situation. This reference guide will provide you everything you need to establish a differential and accurate diagnosis that will lead you to best manage a cardiovascular patient in an emergent situation.

With the first part devoted to basic instrumentation and image acquisition and the second part focusing on the different clinical situations that often require evaluation by echocardiography in the urgent setting, this book is the ideal companion to the physician who needs to implement rapid life and death decisions.

You should use this book as a quick reference guide to echocardiography in the urgent setting. It is designed to help in situations where seconds and minutes can really make a difference in the lives of patients. Even one extra saved life will justify the large amount of work that the authors have put into this work.

Vladimir Fridman and Mario Garcia

Ultrasound physics

Vladimir Fridman

Cardiovascular Diseases, New York, NY, USA

Echocardiography is one of the most valuable diagnostic tests for the evaluation of patients with suspected cardiovascular disease in the acute setting. Even though echocardiography has become more widely available, its performance and interpretation require practice and knowledge of the principles of image formation. Although the physical principles and instrumentation of ultrasound can be quiet complex, there are a few basic concepts that every echocardiographer and interpreting physician must understand to maximize the diagnostic utility of this test and avoid misinterpretations. These key concepts are covered in this chapter.

The echocardiogram machine (Figure 1.1) is made up of few distinct components:

1 Monitor
2 CPU (central processing unit), responsible for all functions of the echocardiogram
3 Transducer
4 Keyboard/controls
5 Printer

The control panel of any echocardiogram looks similar to that shown in Figure 1.2a. The panel is shown in more detail in Figures 1.2b–d, with the important controls labeled. Although slight changes in control positions are noted between machines from different companies, all machines have the key controls that are shown in these images.

The panel from above image, is split into three frames, and the important controls are labeled below.

Practical Manual of Echocardiography in the Urgent Setting, First Edition.
Edited by Vladimir Fridman and Mario J. Garcia.
© 2013 John Wiley & Sons, Ltd. Published 2013 by John Wiley & Sons, Ltd.

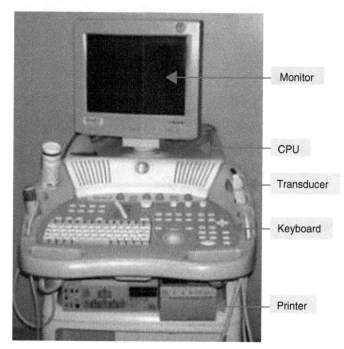

Figure 1.1 Echocardiogram machine.

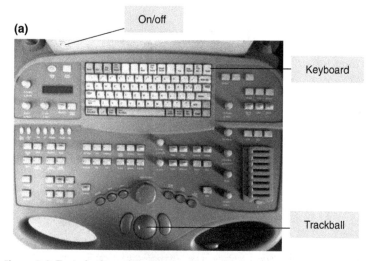

Figure 1.2 Typical echocardiogram control panel.

(b)

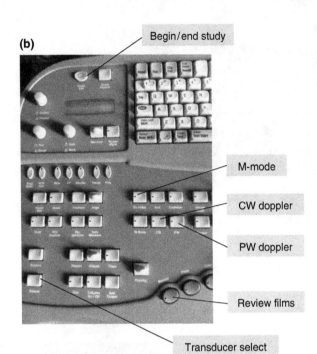

Begin/end study

M-mode

CW doppler

PW doppler

Review films

Transducer select

(c)

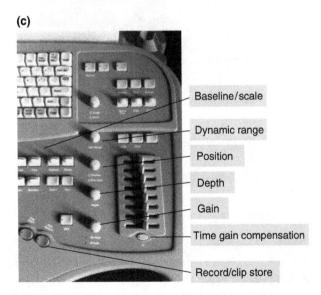

Baseline/scale

Dynamic range

Position

Depth

Gain

Time gain compensation

Record/clip store

Figure 1.2 (*Cont'd*)

(d)

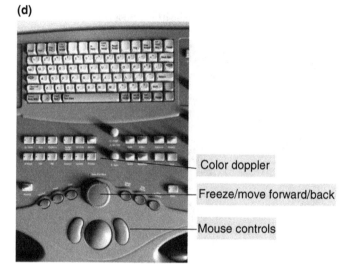

Color doppler

Freeze/move forward/back

Mouse controls

Figure 1.2 (*Cont'd*)

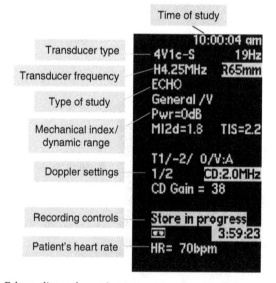

Time of study

Transducer type

Transducer frequency

Type of study

Mechanical index/
dynamic range

Doppler settings

Recording controls

Patient's heart rate

10:00:04 am
4V1c-S   19Hz
H4.25MHz R65mm
ECHO
General /V
Pwr=0dB
MI2d=1.8   TIS=2.2

T1/-2/ 0/V:A
1/2   CD:2.0MHz
CD Gain = 38

Store in progress
[▣]   3:59:23
HR= 70bpm

Figure 1.3 Echocardiography settings.

The important echocardiographic settings as displayed on the monitor of most ultrasound machines are shown in Figure 1.3. These settings can be changed, as needed, to adjust the image quality.

The different echocardiographic modes that are available, which are described later in this book, are:

- M-mode: a graphic representation of a specific line of interest of a two-dimensional image (Figure 1.4).

- 2D: a two-dimensional view of cardiac structures that can be visualized as time progresses (Figure 1.5).
- Color Doppler: a color representation of blood flow velocities superimposed on a two-dimensional image (Figure 1.6).
- CW/PW Doppler: the representation of flow velocities as plotted with time on the x axis and velocity on the y axis (Figure 1.7).
- Tissue Doppler: the measurement of tissue velocities (Figure 1.8).

The controls, as shown in the figures, switch between the different modes of echocardiography. However, before moving on to performing and

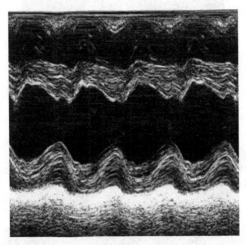

Figure 1.4 M-Mode: a graphic representation of a specific line of interest of a two-dimensional image.

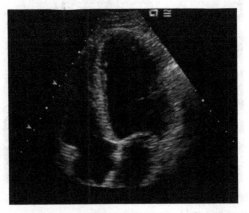

Figure 1.5 2D: a two-dimensional view of cardiac structures that can be visualized as time progresses.

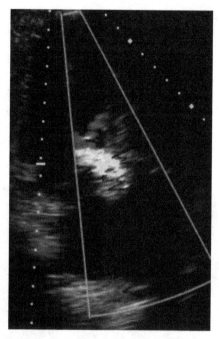

Figure 1.6 Color Doppler: a color representation of blood flow velocities superimposed on a two-dimensional image.

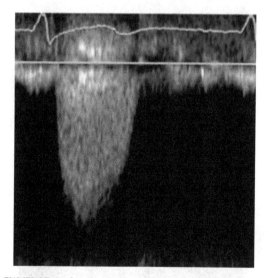

Figure 1.7 CW/PW Doppler: the representation of flow velocities as plotted with time on the x axis and velocity on the y axis.

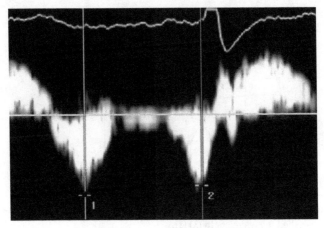

Figure 1.8 Tissue Doppler: the measurement of tissue velocities.

interpreting echocardiograms, it is necessary to be aware of the physics behind this imaging modality.

Ultrasound generation

Ultrasound is a cyclic sound pressure waveform whose frequency is greater than the limit of human hearing. This number is generally considered to be 20 kHz, or 20 000 Hz (Hertz). Echocardiography usually relies on sound waves ranging from 2 to 8 MHz. The echocardiograph, or any other medical ultrasound machine, produces these high frequency sound waves using transducers that contain a piezoelectric crystal.

A piezoelectric crystal (such as quartz or titanate cyramics) is a special material that compresses and expands as electricity is applied to it. This compression and expansion generates the ultrasound wave. The rate (frequency) of compression and expansion is based on the current that the ultrasound machine applies to the piezoelectric signal, which in turn is based on the settings the operator has selected on the machine.

An ultrasound wave, as all sound waves, has some basic physical properties (Figure 1.9). These are:

- Cycle – the sum of one compression and one expansion of a sound wave.
- Frequency (f) – the number of cycles per second.
- Wavelength (λ) – the length of one complete cycle of sound.
- Period (p) – the time duration of one cycle.
- Amplitude – the maximum pressure change from baseline of a sound wave.
- Velocity (v) – speed at which sound moves through a specific medium.

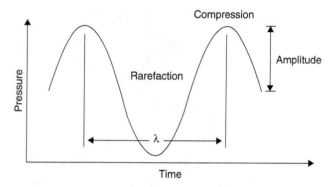

Figure 1.9 A sound wave is made up of varying pressure cycles formed by repeating of compression and rarefaction. The distance between similar points in a wave is called the wavelength (λ) [1].

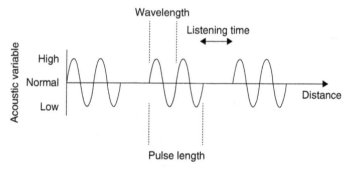

Figure 1.10 A pulse can consist of multiple wavelengths of a sound wave. In this figure, three pulses are shown, each the length of two wavelengths (Reproduced from Case [2], with permisison from Elsevier).

A basic property of all sound waves is: Velocity = Frequency (f) x Wavelength (λ). This formula shows that frequency and wavelength are inversely related, since the velocity of a sound wave depends on the density of the medium the wave is traveling in.

In an echocardiogram machine, current is applied to the piezoelectric crystal, which then emits ultrasound energy into human tissue. The ultrasound is emitted in pulses that usually consist of several consecutive cycles of a sound wave with the same frequency separated by a pause (Figure 1.10). An extremely important concept for ultrasound is the frequency of pulses that the ultrasound emits; this is called the Pulse Repetition Frequency (PRF). The inverse of PRF is the Pulse Repetition Period (PRP), which is the time from the beginning of one ultrasound pulse to the next:

$$PRF = 1 / PRP$$

The actual length of the pulse – the spatial pulse length (SPL) – is equal to the wavelength multiplied by the number of cycles in a pulse.

Once an ultrasound pulse is emitted from the transducer, the entire mechanism enters the "listening" phase. At this time, the ultrasound machine is waiting to receive back the pulse it emitted after it was reflected from distant structures. It is important to know that the ultrasound machine spends almost 99% of the time listening for, and 1% of the time generating, a signal.

Image formation

As the ultrasound wave exits the echocardiogram probe, it enters the human tissue. When the ultrasound waves encounter a change in tissue density, such as the endocardium–blood interphase, some of them will be reflected back while others will penetrate deeper into the tissue. Thus, ultrasound energy is greater near the transducer and is progressively lost as it penetrates into the tissue. The ultrasound systems typically compensate by amplifying more the signals that are received from the far field to make the image homogeneous. The interaction of ultrasound with human tissue is also very complex. However, it is important to know that within soft tissue the velocity of ultrasound is fairly constant at 1540 m/s. In fact, it is usually assumed that this is the velocity of sound in human tissue. However, it is not always the truth. The velocities of ultrasound in various human tissues are shown in Table 1.1.

This concept is extremely important, since the ultrasound machine is not able to recognize whether the ultrasound it receives back from the body traveled mainly through bone, through soft tissue, through air, or any combination of the above structures. As such, it computes the distance the ultrasound traveled based on a velocity of 1540 m/s. Therefore, objects can be misplaced on an ultrasound image because of this velocity assumption, which is built into the ultrasound machine. This explains

Table 1.1 Velocity of ultrasound in various human tissues.

Medium	Velocity (m/s)
Air (the slowest)	330
Soft tissue	1540
Blood	1570
Muscle	1580
Bone (the fastest)	4080

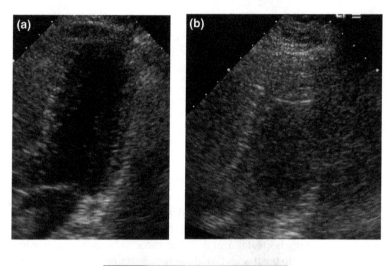

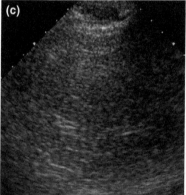

Figure 1.11 An apical four-chamber view of the same patient when the patient has exhaled **(a)**, as the patient is inhaling **(b)**, and as the patient is fully inhaled **(c)**. As clearly seen, the quality of the myocardial image declines acutely as more air enters the lung of the patient, to a point where no myocardium is seen in full inhalation **(c)**.

why interposition of ribs or lung tissue between the transducer and the heart will produce severe imaging artifacts and make part of the image uninterpretable (Figure 1.11).

Another important point to remember is the behavior of the ultrasound beam as it emerges from the transducer (Figure 1.12). The ultrasound beam is initially parallel and cylindrical (near zone). However, after its narrowest point, the focal zone, it begins to diverge and acquires a cone shape (far zone). For reasons outside the scope of this book, the imaging is much better if the object of interest is located near the focal zone. The near zone length is calculated via: near field = (radius of transducer)^2/wavelength of ultrasound. The location of the focal zone can be adjusted electronically.

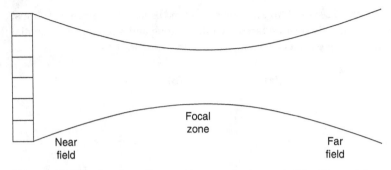

Figure 1.12 Behavior of an ultrasound beam as it comes out of the ultrasound probe (Reproduced from [2] Case, TD. Ultrasound Physics and Instrumentation. Surg Clinc N Am. 1998;78(2):197–217).

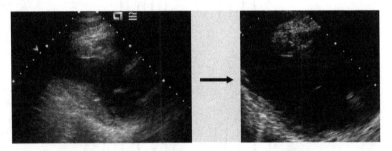

Figure 1.13 Image changes with a decrease in ultrasound frequency.

Resolution versus penetration

The behavior of the beam within tissue determines the lateral resolution of the ultrasound, or the ability to distinguish two objects located side by side on an ultrasound image. The axial resolution, or the ability to distinguish two objects one in front of the other, on an ultrasound image is determined by ultrasound transducer frequency (1/wavelength). At higher frequency, axial resolution increases. However, since the ultrasound signal is attenuated as it travels through the tissues, more attenuation occurs. In general, high frequency is preferred for imaging structures that are closer to the transducer and lower frequency for those that are far. In the case shown in Figure 1.13, a parasternal long axis view loses its definition as the transducer frequency is changed from 4.0 MHz to 2.0 MHz.

As the ultrasound comes back to the transducer, the same piezoelectric properties of crystal that allow the ultrasound waves to be made allow the conversion of the received ultrasound waves into electrical signals. A typical 2D ultrasound transducer has 128 or 256 individual crystal-electronic interphases. In M-mode imaging, the ultrasound beam is emitted and received only at 90°. By alternating the time and sequence in which these are stimulated, the ultrasound beam can be steered at almost any angle. By steering rapidly while emitting and receiving at sequential angles a two-dimensional image is formed (Figure 1.14).

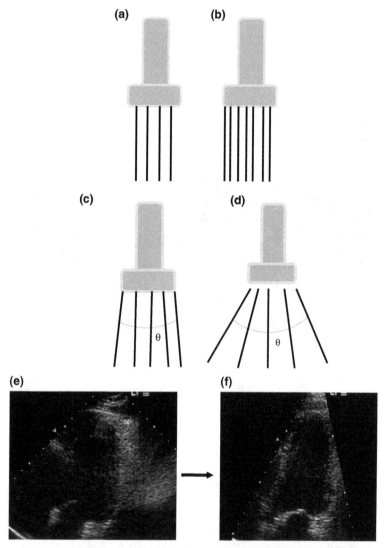

Figure 1.14 As the scan line density increases (**a**→**b**), the accuracy and resolution of the image increase. As the sector angle (θ) increases (**c**→**d**), more structures are noted as the area being interrogated by the ultrasound beam increases. However, going to a narrower angle (**e**→**f**) increases resolution, as is seen in this set of images where a wider view (**e**) shows multiple structures, while the same view with a narrower sector angle (**f**) more clearly shows the endocardial definition of the left ventricle.

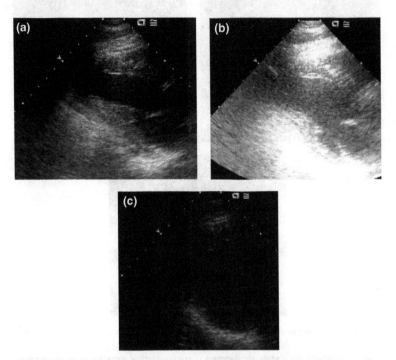

Figure 1.15 Effect of changing the gain settings on echocardiographic images.

Important controls of 2D image formation are:
- Scan line density – the number of distinct scan lines per unit area of image. The higher the number, the more accurate the image.
- Sector angle – the angle at which image acquisition takes place. The larger the angle, the more structures are visualized in the image, but the slower image acquisition takes place.
- Imaging depth – the depth of structures that are visualized in the image. The larger the depth, the longer it takes for the ultrasound to receive the reflected ultrasound waves from those structures, and the slower the image acquisition occurs.

Additional parameters that should be adjusted during M-mode and 2D examination include:
- Gain – the intensity of recorded signal. Figure 1.15 shows the effects of increasing gain (a→b) and decreasing gain (a→c).
- Dynamic range – the range of lowest and highest intensity signals recorded. Figure 1.16 shows the effects of increasing dynamic range (a→b) and decreasing dynamic range (a→c).
- Time–Gain Compensation (TGC) – the increasing or decreasing of signal strength due to depth of the structure that it is reflected from. TGC can be used to strengthen the proximal structures (Figure 1.17b)

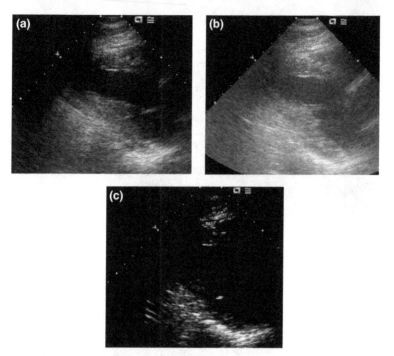

Figure 1.16 Effect of changing the dynamic range on echocardiographic images.

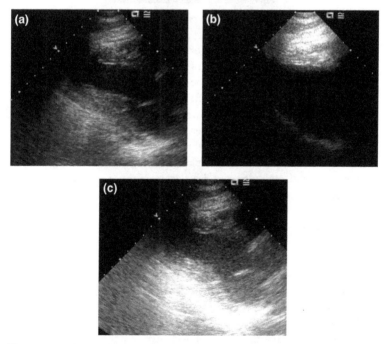

Figure 1.17 Effect of changing the Time-Gain Compensation on echocardiographic images.

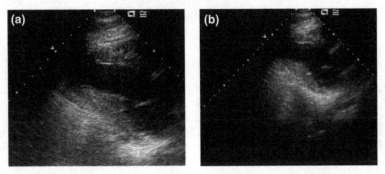

Figure 1.18 Effect of changing the depth on echocardiographic images.

or the distal structures (Figure 1.17c), when compared to baseline image (Figure 1.17a).

- Depth – the length of tissue penetration that is recorded in an image. Increasing the depth will allow the visualization of more distal structures (Figure 1.18a→b).
- Sweep rate (M-mode only) – the speed of the M-mode image as it is displayed on the monitor.

Doppler ultrasound

Doppler images are generated based on a different set of physical principles. The frequency of an ultrasound wave changes slightly when reflected by an object that is either approaching (increasing), or moving away (decreasing), from the source of the wave (Figure 1.19a). This is applied in echocardiography to measure the velocity of a moving column of blood or the myocardium itself (tissue Doppler). When the reflected waves return back to the ultrasound probe, the change in frequency detected allows the echocardiograph to determine the velocity of the moving reflector. A major limitation of Doppler imaging is that, for it to be accurate, the reflector should be traveling in a parallel direction to the ultrasound wave. If the reflector travels at an angle, only the parallel component of the vector of motion is detected. If the angle of travel is known, the velocity of travel of the reflector can be determined by multiplying the parallel component measured by the ultrasound system by the cosine of the angle of incidence (Figure 1.19b). However, when the direction of travel cannot be determined, significant underestimation can occur when the object is moving at an angle that exceeds 20°.

The Doppler shift equation, as applied to echocardiography, is:

$$\Delta F = (Fr - Ft) = (2Ft\, V \cos \theta)/C$$

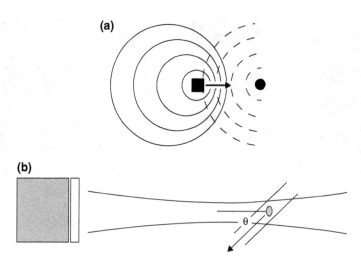

Figure 1.19 The frequency of a wave changes as it approaches, or moves away, from a stationary object **(a)**. The accuracy of Doppler to record a change in frequency depends on the angle of intersection (θ) between the Doppler beam and the flow of blood **(b)** (Reproduced from Coltrera [1], with permission from Elsevier).

where ΔF=change in frequency, Ft=transmitted frequency, Fr=reflected frequency, V=velocity of blood moving toward the transducer, C=velocity of sound in tissue, and θ=angle between sound beam and direction of blood flow.

In echocardiography, there are two major types of Doppler modes used: Continuous Wave (CW) Doppler and Pulsed Wave (PW) Doppler.

Continuous Wave (CW) Doppler is the older and electronically simpler of the two types of Doppler. It involves continuous generation of ultrasound waves by the transducer and continuous reception of ultrasound waves by the transducer. It requires at least a two crystal transducer, with one crystal devoted to each of the functions. Because in CW Doppler ultrasound the ultrasound waves are sent continuously, more waves are sent in a given period of time and the receiver can detect larger shifts in frequency, thus providing a higher range of velocity resolution. At the same time, since there are no pauses between ultrasound pulses, the receiver cannot determine the pulse travel time, and thus cannot localize the depth of reflectors. If there are several objects moving at different velocities across the path of the ultrasound beam, the transducer will record multiple frequency shifts, producing a dense spectral image where only the maximum velocity can be identified.

Pulsed Wave (PW) Doppler involves a transducer that alternates between sending and receiving the ultrasound waves. Because less ultrasound waves

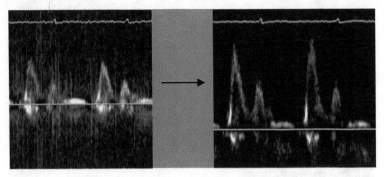

Figure 1.20 Adjustment of sample volume prevents Doppler artifacts.

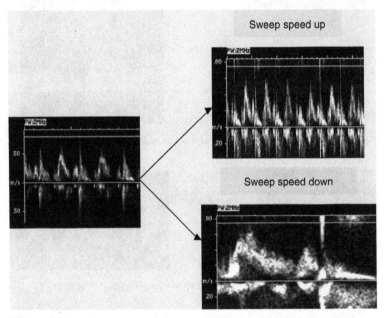

Figure 1.21 Effect of changing the sweep speed on echocardiographic images.

are sent in a given period of time the maximum frequency shift that can be detected is limited but the depth where the velocity shift occurs may be determined by measuring the travel time of the ultrasound pulses.

Parameters that should be adjusted during Doppler examination include:

- Sample volume (pulse mode only) – placement of the sample volume in the exact location of the needed measurement prevents artifacts and other flows from interfering with Doppler imaging (Figure 1.20).
- Doppler gain – the intensity of the incoming signal that gets recorded as a separate signal.

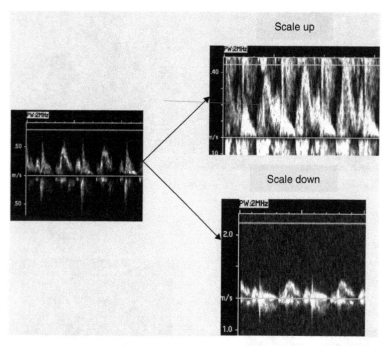

Figure 1.22 Effect of changing the scale on echocardiographic images.

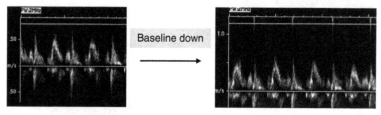

Figure 1.23 Effect of shifting the baseline on echocardiographic images.

- Sweep rate – the speed at which the resulting image moves across the screen (Figure 1.21).
- Scale – the amount of space on the monitor screen corresponding to a specific unit of measurement (Figure 1.22).
- Baseline – the velocity recorded as zero or no flow (Figure 1.23).

Aliasing is a phenomenon that occurs when the object being interrogated by PW Doppler is moving faster than the maximum velocity the PW can interrogate (Nyquist limit). The resulting image places portion of the Doppler image above the baseline, and a portion wraps around and starts below the baseline (Figure 1.24). This image is uninterpretable and CW should be used instead in this case.

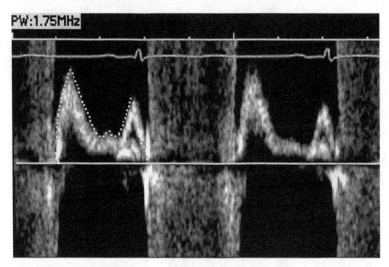

Figure 1.24 PW Doppler of the mitral flow. The mitral regurgitation jet is seen aliasing.

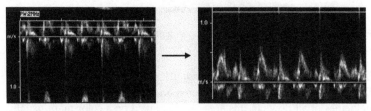

Figure 1.25 Aliasing of the mitral inflow on the left-hand image is fixed by a lower baseline on the right-hand image.

The mathematical principle behind aliasing is complex. However, it is important to know that it depends on the pulse repetition frequency (PRF), which is determined by the interval between pulses. The maximum velocity that can be interrogated by PW is PRF/2. However, the Nyquist limit can be increased in one direction by shifting the baseline in the opposite direction. For example, if the velocity of the flow of interest exceeds the Nyquist limit and the reflector is moving away from the transducer, the Nyquist limit may be increased by shifting the baseline (Figure 1.25).

For a novice echocardiographer, it is always hard to determine whether to use PW or CW for interrogation of specific flows. As a quick rule, major stenotic and regurgitant lesions should be interrogated with CW, but flows that need to be interrogated at a specific location should be interrogated with PW.

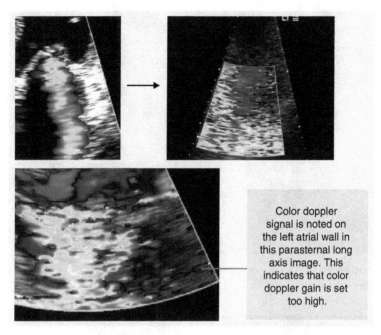

Color doppler signal is noted on the left atrial wall in this parasternal long axis image. This indicates that color doppler gain is set too high.

Figure 1.26 Effect of changing the Doppler gain on echocardiographic images.

Another important Doppler modality is color Doppler. When color Doppler is used to interrogate an area on a two-dimensional image, the velocities of all flows in this area are displayed on a color map (usually, red represents movement toward the transducer and blue away from the transducer). The colors represent the velocities of flow at the point in which the color is displayed. This type of imaging is very frequently used to visualize regurgitant and turbulent flows within all the structures of the heart. Parameters that require adjustment in color Doppler are:

- Color maps – the specific colors assigned to flow toward and away from the transducer.
- Sector – the area to be interrogated by color Doppler. The smaller the area, the more accurate the signal.
- Gain – the frequency of the reflected signal that is reported on a color map. As shown in Figure 1.26, a lot of artifacts are created when the color Doppler is overgained. Here, a moderate to severe MR signal is turned into an interpretable image when the color Doppler gain is increased fully. The golden rule is that color Doppler gain should be set to a setting just below the level at which speckles of color Doppler signal are seen in the background images (such as on the myocardium itself, where no flow is occurring).

- Scale – the range of velocities interpreted by color Doppler. Set by pulse repetition frequency (PFR).
- Baseline – the velocity that is considered to have zero or no flow. Changing this setting will alter the range of velocities that are displayed on the color Doppler screen (Figure 1.27).

Tissue Doppler uses the basic Doppler principles to record myocardial tissue velocities. It is very useful in evaluating myocardial systolic and diastolic function. It may be applied in pulsed or color modes.

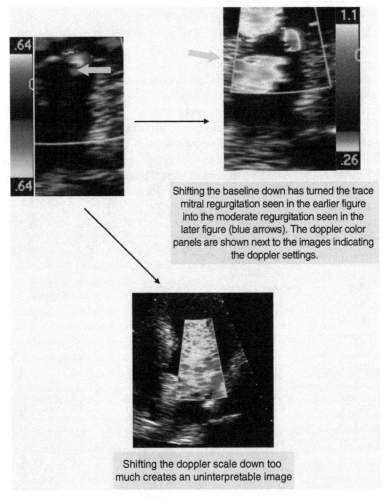

Shifting the baseline down has turned the trace mitral regurgitation seen in the earlier figure into the moderate regurgitation seen in the later figure (blue arrows). The doppler color panels are shown next to the images indicating the doppler settings.

Shifting the doppler scale down too much creates an uninterpretable image

Figure 1.27 Effect of changing the color Doppler baseline on echocardiographic images.

Summary and key points

Echocardiography is a very powerful tool that may be used to evaluate cardiac anatomy and function in the acute setting, However, not everything that is seen on an ultrasound image represents a real finding. Ultrasound images contain both true anatomical and functional information as well as artifacts produced by the interaction between ultrasound waves and the medium. Proper understanding of basic ultrasound principles and optimal adjustment of the instrument settings can dramatically improve image quality and the likelihood of providing accurate and complete diagnostic information.

When conducting an ultrasound examination:

1 Record name, medical record and other demographic information properly.
2 Close windows and dim lights.
3 Position the patient and request his/her cooperation during image acquisition.
4 Remove unnecessary clothing and cables.
5 Place ECG leads and verify adequate recording.
6 Set up digital and acquisition parameters (ECG triggered versus time triggered, number of loops).
7 Select appropriate transducer and apply abundant conducting gel.
8 Select appropriate protocols/machine set-up.
9 Follow a standard acquisition protocol.
10 Optimize gain, dynamic range (contrast), TGCs, imaging frequency, depth, filters, scales for every view.
11 Verify that data are properly stored.

If image quality is difficult:

• Reposition patient.
• Seek alternative imaging windows.
• Re-apply gel.
• Re-adjust frequency, gain and other parameters.

References

1 Coltrera, MD. Ultrasound Physics in a Nutshell. *Otolaryngol Clin N Am* 2010; 43:1149–59.
2 Case, TD. Ultrasound Physics and Instrumentation. *Surg Clin N Am* 1998;78(2): 197–217.

The transthoracic examination

Vladimir Fridman[1] and Dennis Finkielstein[2]

[1]Cardiovascular Diseases, New York, NY, USA
[2]Beth Israel Medical Center and Albert Einstein College of Medicine, New York, NY, USA

CHAPTER 2

During transthoracic echocardiography (TTE) the ultrasound probe is applied to multiple points on the patient's chest and images are taken of all cardiac structures from multiple tomographic planes (Table 2.1). Before starting the procedure is important to verify that the correct patient information is entered in the ultrasound machine, the correct presets for transthoracic imaging are selected, the patient is position whenever possible in the left lateral decubitus, the chest is exposed and the ECG leads are properly placed.

The 2011 ACCF/ASE/AHA/ASNC/HFSA/HRS/SCAI/SCCM/SCCT/SCMR 2011 Appropriateness Use Criteria for Echocardiography listed appropriate, uncertain, and inappropriate reasons for the use of echocardiography (Box 2.1)[1].

The indications for an "emergency echocardiogram" differ from those of a routine examination.

Although the main indications for an emergency echocardiography are shown in Box 2.1, it is reasonable to perform a TTE whenever the results could lead to change in treatment in a critically ill patient, irrespective of the indication.

Two types of TTE may be performed in the acute setting:

1 Complete – includes all views, Doppler measurements, and appropriate calculations.

2 Limited – covers only the important structures, such as ruling out pericardial effusion.

As a goal, unless timing does not allow, a complete echocardiogram should be performed at all times.

Practical Manual of Echocardiography in the Urgent Setting, First Edition.
Edited by Vladimir Fridman and Mario J. Garcia.
© 2013 John Wiley & Sons, Ltd. Published 2013 by John Wiley & Sons, Ltd.

Table 2.1 Standard echocardiographic views.

Parasternal window	Apical window	Subcostal window
Long Axis	4-chamber view	4-chamber view
RV inflow view	2-chamber view	5-chamber view
RV outflow view	3-chamber view	Short axis view
Short axis at mitral valve	5-chamber view	Inferior Vena Cava view
Short axis at papillary muscles		
Short axis at base		
Short axis at aortic valve		
Suprasternal notch views are used to visualize the aortic arch and other nearby structures		

Box 2.1 Indications for emergency echocardiography

1 Hemodynamic compromise.
2 Suspected acute MI. However, a TTE should never delay a catheterization in setting of STEMI.
3 New heart failure presentation.
4 Cases where pericardial effusion/cardiac tamponade are part of the differential diagnosis.
5 New murmur, especially in setting of new cardiac symptoms.
6 Acute onset of cardiac symptoms.
7 Chest pain without a definitive ECG and/or cardiac biomarkers.
8 Change in patient status post procedures (cardiac or noncardiac).

It is important to know what the indication for the echocardiogram is prior to starting the test and the clinical status of the patient, as well as to consider a differential diagnosis. This is especially important for urgent/emergent studies since, if time is of the essence, specific views will be prioritized and the clinical question can be appropriately answered as soon as possible.

A complete echocardiogram includes all of the views listed in Table 2.1. The pertinent structures seen in the 2D TTE views shown below.

• Parasternal long axis view (Figure 2.1)
  ○ Left ventricle (LV): global and regional wall motion assessment
  ○ Mitral valve and mitral valve apparatus
  ○ Left atrium (LA)
  ○ LV outflow tract (LVOT)
  ○ Aortic valve

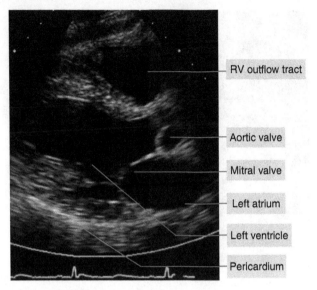

RV outflow tract

Aortic valve

Mitral valve

Left atrium

Left ventricle

Pericardium

Figure 2.1 Parasternal long axis view.

- ○ Aortic root and proximal portion of ascending aorta
- ○ Often, the right pulmonary artery is seen in this view – it is normally physically close to, and is 90° apart in axis from, the ascending aorta
- ○ Right ventricle outflow tract (RVOT) – it is important to note that the main body of the RV is not seen in this view
- ○ Descending aorta – normally in cross section
- ○ Coronary sinus
- ○ Pericardium
- ○ Of note – the apex of the heart should not be seen in this view. If thought to be visualized, the image is foreshortened and a better view should be obtained for analysis.
- • RV inflow view (Figure 2.2)
  - ○ Right ventricle
  - ○ Right atrium
  - ○ Tricuspid valve: Posterior and septal leaflets – this is the only standard view where the posterior leaflet of the tricuspid valve is visualized; all other views have anterior and septal leaflets
  - ○ Inferior vena cava (IVC).
- • RV outflow view (Figure 2.3)
  - ○ Right ventricle
  - ○ Pulmonary artery: with bifurcation into the right and left main pulmonary arteries
  - ○ Tricuspid valve.

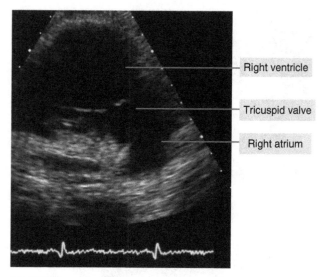

Figure 2.2 RV inflow view.

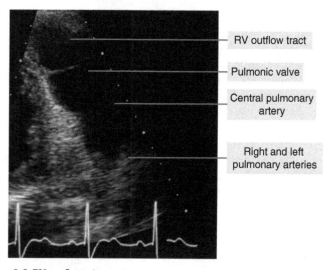

Figure 2.3 RV outflow view.

- Parasternal short axis view at mitral valve and papillary muscle levels (Figure 2.4 and 2.5).
  - ○ LV cavity
  - ○ Mitral valve, if taken at mitral valve level
  - ○ Posteromedial and anterolateral papillary muscles, if taken at the papillary muscle level.

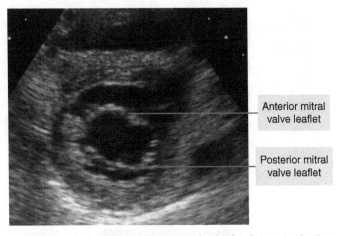

Figure 2.4 Parasternal short axis view at mitral valve level. Anterior (top) and posterior (bottom) leaflet of the mitral valve is noted.

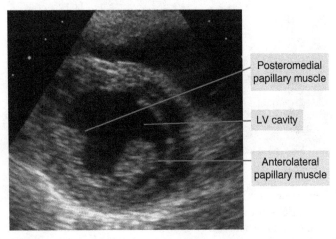

Figure 2.5 Parasternal short axis view at papillary muscle level. Anterolateral (right side of the picture) and posteromedial (left side of the picture) papillary muscles are seen in this view.

- Parasternal short axis view at aortic valve level (at the base) (Figure 2.6)
  - Right atrium
  - Right ventricle
  - RVOT
  - Pulmonic valve
  - Pulmonary artery
  - Aortic valve – all three cusps (left, right, and noncoronary); as a rule, the noncoronary cusp is always the closest cusp to the interatrial septum

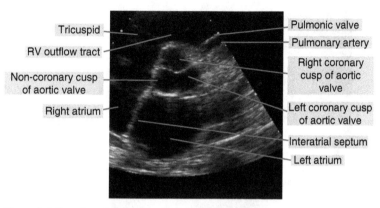

Figure 2.6 Parasternal short axis view at the base.

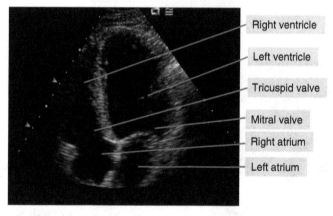

Figure 2.7 Apical four-chamber view.

- ○ Left atrium
- ○ Interatrial septum.
- • Apical four-chamber view (Figure 2.7)
  - ○ LV wall segments, as shown in Figure 2.8
  - ○ Mitral valve
  - ○ Tricuspid valve – as a general rule, the tricuspid valve is positioned more apically than the mitral valve
  - ○ Right ventricle
  - ○ Left atrium
  - ○ Right atrium
  - ○ Pulmonary veins are often visualized coming into the LA.
- • Apical five-chamber view (Figure 2.9)
  - ○ LV wall segments, as shown in Figure 2.8
  - ○ Structures similar to apical four-chamber view
  - ○ LVOT

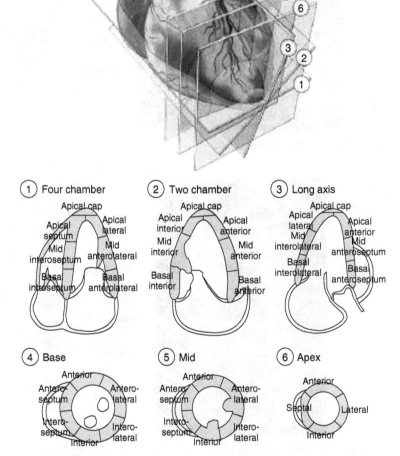

Figure 2.8 The 17-segment nomeclature model of LV wall segments, as seen in multiple echocardiographic views (Reproduced from [2], with permission from Elsevier).

- ○ Aortic valve
- ○ Proximal ascending aorta
- ○ The Pedoff (nonimaging) probe should be used in the apical position in cases of possible aortic stenosis

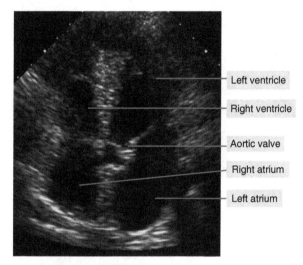

Figure 2.9 Apical five-chamber view.

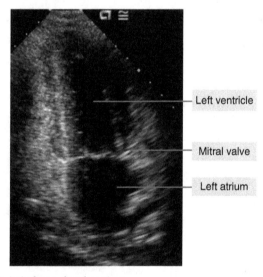

Figure 2.10 Apical two-chamber view

- Apical two-chamber view (Figure 2.10)
  - LV wall segments, as shown in Figure 2.8
  - Mitral valve
  - Left atrium
  - Occasionally, the left atrial appendage can be visualized
  - Coronary sinus.

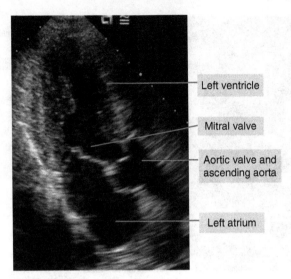

Left ventricle

Mitral valve

Aortic valve and
ascending aorta

Left atrium

Figure 2.11 Apical three-chamber view.

- Apical three-chamber view – also known as apical long axis view (Figure 2.11)
  - LV wall segments, as shown in Figure 2.8
  - Mitral valve
  - Aortic valve
  - Proximal ascending aorta.
- Subcostal four-chamber view (Figure 2.12)
  - LV wall segments, as shown in Figure 2.8
  - Right ventricle
  - Left atrium
  - Right atrium
  - Interatrial septum – this is a good view to perform an agitated saline contrast study to check for patent foramen ovale (PFO)/atrial septal defect (ASD).
- Subcostal five-chamber view
  - Structures appearing in the subcostal four-chamber view plus:
  - LVOT
  - Aortic valve
  - Proximal ascending aorta.
- Subcostal short axis view
  - As in apical short axis view, the structures seen in this view depend on what level of the heart the view taken
  - The actual structures seen are similar to the structures seen in the apical short axis.

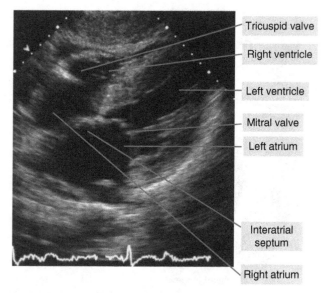

Figure 2.12 Subcostal four-chamber view.

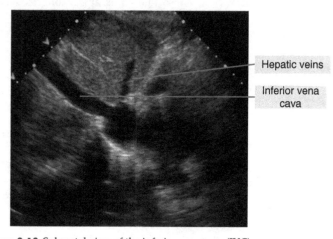

Figure 2.13 Subcostal view of the inferior vena cava (IVC).

- Subcostal inferior vena cava view (Figure 2.13)
  - Inferior vena cava
  - Hepatic veins
  - Eustachian valve and, if present, the Chiari Network
  - It is important to make sure when measuring the IVC that it is the actual IVC that is being measured. Many novice operators will measure one of the hepatic veins as the IVC. To make sure the

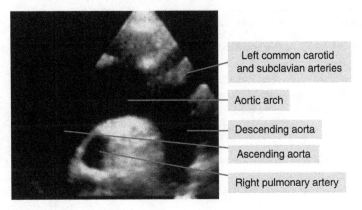

Left common carotid and subclavian arteries

Aortic arch

Descending aorta

Ascending aorta

Right pulmonary artery

Figure 2.14 Suprasternal notch view (Reproduced from Schwammenthal *et al.* [3], with permission from Elsevier).

actual IVC is in view, it should be traced from its drainage point into the right atrium all throughout the view. It should also not have branches or splitting points within the liver.

- Suprasternal notch view (Figure 2.14)
  - ○ Ascending aorta
  - ○ Aortic arch
  - ○ Descending aorta
  - ○ Brachiocephalic artery
  - ○ Left subclavian artery
  - ○ Left common carotid artery
  - ○ This view can be used to look for an aortic coarctation or dissection
  - ○ A Pedoff probe should be used from this view in cases of possible aortic stenosis.

As an echocardiogram is performed, it is important to pay attention to all of the walls of the left ventricle in all of the different views. The most recent, 17-segment, model of LV wall nomeclature is shown in Figure 2.8.

Performing the echocardiogram

Whether performing an elective, complete echocardiogram, or an emergent, limited echocardiogram, it is still vital to try to position the patient properly and adjust the environment around the patient to yield the best possible echocardiography windows/images (Boxes 2.2 and 2.3).

It is especially important to:

Box 2.2 Steps involved in preparing the patient

1 Inform the patient about the procedure.
2 Have the patient take off their sweater/shirt or undo the hospital gown so that the entire chest is available for the imaging procedure.
3 Remove any unused electrodes from the patient's chest.
4 If possible, have the patient lie in the left lateral decubitus position. In the ICU, a pillow can be placed under the patient's ride side to help with positioning.
5 Attach the echocardiogram machine ECG electrodes to the patient. This is needed for rhythm strip acquisition during echocardiography.
6 Place towel under the left side of the patient to prevent gel from staining the bed/patient.

Box 2.3 Major steps involved in preparing the environment for echocardiography

1 Dim all possible lights.
2 Make as much space as possible in the room for the echocardiogram machine and yourself.
3 Adjust the bed/stretcher in a way to minimize straining yourself.
4 Make sure you have all necessary equipment for the procedure: echocardiogram machine, ECG leads and electrodes, imaging transducer, and liberal amounts of ultrasound gel.

- Spend some extra time preparing the patient and the environment. This will make a lot of difference in the quality of the images you acquire.
- Make sure you adjust the patient and the environment so you are comfortable doing the procedure. One common cause of disability in people performing echocardiograms is repetitive strain injuries. Take the time to adjust the situation so you are comfortable!
- Use as much gel as necessary. As discussed in the Chapter 1, ultrasound is highly attenuated in air. Therefore, the more gel you use, the less the risk there is of attenuation.
- One element of debate in echocardiography involves determining on which side of the patient the echocardiographer should be positioned. The choice of left-hand versus right-hand scanning is a matter of preference, hand dominance and comfort. Nevertheless, it is advisable to learn to scan with both hands. In the critical care setting it may be difficult to scan from the left side or the right side of the patient depending on the specific circumstances and room set-up.

Using the transducer

The M-mode and 2D images in echocardiography are performed with a standard cardiac imaging transducer. The usual frequency range for intracardiac imaging is approximately 2–6 MHz.

Remember:
- The higher the frequency, the better the resolution.
- The lower the frequency, the better the penetration.

For each patient (depending on body mass index, fat deposition, etc.), multiple frequencies should be tried and the one that yields the best image should be used.

Probe manipulations

The four manipulations possible with an echocardiogram probe are [4]:

1 Pressure – the amount of pressure the echocardiographer puts on the patient's chest with the ultrasound probe (Figure 2.15). This maneuver is able to produce some differences in image quality, as putting firm pressure on the transducer can bring it closer to the structure of interest by displacing/compressing fat layers. However, using pressure with the ultrasound probe is uncomfortable for, and might end up with some hostility from, the patient.

2 Alignment – the sonographer's wrist moves left to right, or right to left. The process by which the ultrasound probe is moved on the patient's chest from position to position to bring the object of interest into the field of view (Figure 2.16). Switching the position of the transducer from the parasternal long axis position to the apical four-chamber position to image the apex of the heart is an example of probe alignment.

3 Rotation – clockwise or counterclockwise rotation of the probe. The movement of the ultrasound probe along its long axis. If placed perpendicular to the patient's chest, the transducer can be rotated the full 360° (Figure 2.17). Although, of course, unique imaging planes are only possible up to 180° and, if rotated beyond that point, will produce a "mirror image" to prior views.

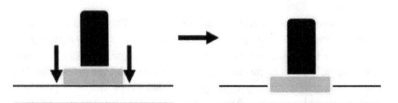

Figure 2.15 In this figure, more pressure is added to the probe, resulting in the probe going deeper into the skin.

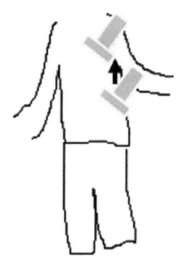

Figure 2.16 In this figure, moving the probe along the chest allows for better alignment with the image of interest.

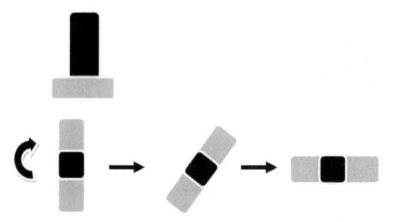

Figure 2.17 A view of the echocardiography probe from below shows the probe being rotated clockwise 90°.

4 Tilt – sonographer's wrist flexes or extends. This implies changing the incline of the ultrasound probe in relation to the patient's chest (Figure 2.18). Usually starting perpendicular to the skin (90˚), lowering or increasing this angle without any movements of the probe along its axis will produce different images and change the shape/appearance of visualized structures. Also, tilting in specific positions can produce totally different views as in going from parasternal long axis view to the RV inflow and outflow views.

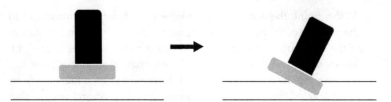

Figure 2.18 In this figure, a probe is being tilted to produce a better image.

Steps involved in a comprehensive transthoracic echocardiogram

1 For the parasternal views, position the probe in the left parasternal space (approximately 2–3 inches to the left of the sternum), between the second and fourth intercostal space. For the parasternal long axis view, the transducer indicator or "notch" should be pointed toward the right shoulder.

   a Slight movements of the transducer as described above, along with movements up and down within the intercostal space, should be performed to optimize the image.

   b In this view:

     i All appropriate structures should be visualized.

     ii M-mode images should be taken at the left ventricle between the mitral valve leaflets and the papillary muscles, mitral valve, and aortic valve leaflet levels.

     iii Color Doppler should be used to quickly interrogate the mitral and aortic valves.

     iv Presence or absence of pericardial effusion should be noted.

2 After the parasternal long axis view, tilting the probe downwards (pointing towards the patient's right hip) will produce the RV inflow view. It is important to not move the ultrasound transducer at this point, just to tilt.

   a This is a hard view to obtain, especially for the novice echocardiographer.

   b However, if obtained, this is a great view to measure the tricuspid regurgitation jet velocity by interrogating the tricuspid valve (this is discussed further in later chapters).

3 Tilting the probe upward (pointing toward the patient's left shoulder) will produce the RV outflow view), and the tricuspid valve can be zoomed on for a closer evaluation.

   a This is also a difficult view to obtain.

   b If obtained, the pulmonic valve can be interrogated. A great view of the pulmonary artery may be obtained in this view.

4 At this point, the echocardiographer should bring the transducer to the position of the parasternal long axis view. A 90° clockwise rotation of the transducer, bringing the transducer notch to point toward the left shoulder, will bring into view the parasternal short axis view.
   a Sweeping the transducer up and down will change the view from the level of the apex, mid-LV cavity, mitral valve, and aortic valve views.
   b To make sure the transducer is positioned correctly, at the level of the mid-LV cavity, the LV walls should form a circle. If the LV cavity is not circular, slight adjustments to the transducer position should be made to correct the view.
5 The next set of views is obtained from the apical window. The true position for these views is located by placing the transducer at the point of maximal impulse. Ordinarily, the fourth or fifth intercostal space, slightly lateral to the nipple.
   a Again, slight movements of the transducer and, if needed, change of the intercostal space, should be performed to visualize the LV along its long axis.
6 To obtain the apical four-chamber view, place the probe at the point of maximal impulse with the notch at the three o'clock position.
7 To obtain the apical five-chamber view, tilting of the probe upward will bring out the anterior structures, such as the LVOT, aortic valve, and proximal ascending aorta. This makes the apical five-chamber view.
8 To obtain the apical two-chamber view, the probe then should be tilted back to its four-chamber view position. An approximately 90° counterclockwise rotation of the probe will produce the apical two-chamber view.
9 To obtain the apical three-chamber view, continued counterclockwise rotation of the probe for a further 60–90° from the apical two-chamber view will result in the apical three-chamber view.
10 After the apical views are obtained, the next step is to attempt the sub-costal view. At this point, the patient should be placed in the supine position. The patient's legs should be bent at the knees with their feet on the stretcher. The patient's head should be slightly elevated.
   a The transducer should be placed in the subxiphoid position. It should be pointed toward the heart. The transducer notch should be pointed to the left side of the patient.
   b Slight movements should be made to align the image with the structures of interest.
11 Counterclockwise rotation of the probe (approximately 90°) from the sub-costal long axis view will yield subcostal short axis view. Tilting manipulations similar to the parasternal short axis view manipulations will bring into view different levels of imaging of the short axis of the heart.

12 Tilting the probe fully to the right, thus aligning the beam with the liver, without changing the position of the probe on the patient's chest, should bring into view the liver and the IVC.

   a This manipulation is difficult, especially for the novice echocardiographer. However, slight movements of the probe as it is pointed toward the liver usually bring the correct view.

   b As discussed previously, it is important to make sure that the structure being imaged is the IVC and not the hepatic veins, since IVC measurements are extremely useful in an echocardiogram (this is discussed in later chapters).

13 The final view is the suprasternal view. The patient should be lying flat on the back, facing toward the left side, and with the chin lifted upward. The probe is positioned in the suprasternal notch. The transducer notch is pointed toward the left side of the patient.

   a The ultrasound probe should be slightly tilted upward and downward until the best view is obtained.

   b As described above, this is a great view to look for an aortic coarctation.

After the echocardiogram is complete, a report is made and finalized in a timely fashion. If it is an urgent/emergent study, a preliminary report should be put into the chart immediately after the study, and a final report should be made as soon as possible. If it is an elective echocardiogram, a report should simply be made as soon as possible.

Important parts of preliminary and final reports are listed in Box 2.4 [5].

Box 2.4 Basic report elements

Name of patient
Medical record number and/or Date of birth
Date of study
Time of study and of preliminary report
Indication for study
Report must mention all pertinent positive and negative findings, such as:
  Assessment of LV function
  Assessment of RV function
  Presence/absence of wall motion abnormalities
  Description of the aorta, main pulmonary artery and IVC
  Any pertinent hemodynamic data
  Presence/absence of pericardial effusion
  Valvular structure/function and any stenosis/regurgitation (all valves)
  Any other findings pertinent to clinical situation

It should be noted that all preliminary reports should state that this is a preliminary report and that a final report is pending and is going to be reported separately.

In most circumstances, a note should be left in the medical record indicating that the procedure was completed. This note must include the time of completion, the name of the individual who performed the study and a phone number where a preliminary report could be obtained. Critical results should always be communicated to the ordering physician immediately.

References

1 Echocardiographic writing group. Appropriate use criteria for echocardiography. *J Am Soc Echocardiogr* 2011; 24:229–67.
2 Chamber Quantification Writing Group. Recommendations for Chamber Quantification: A Report from the American Society of Echocardiography's Guidelines and Standards Committee and the Chamber Quantification Writing Group, Developed in Conjunction with the European Association of Echocardiography, a Branch of the European Society of Cardiology. *J Am Soc Echocardiogr* 2005; 18:1440–63.
3 Schwammenthal E, Schwammenthal Y, Tanne D, *et al.* Transcutaneous detection of aortic arch atheromas by suprasternal harmonic imaging. *J Am Coll Cardiol* 2002; 39(7):1127–32.
4 Ihnatsenka B and Boezaart AP. Ultrasound: Basic understanding and learning the language. *Int J Shoulder Surg* 2010; 4(3): 55–62.
5 Picard MH, Adams D, Bierig SM, *et al.* American Society of Echocardiography recommendations for quality echocardiography laboratory operation. *J Am Soc Echocardiogr* 2011; 24(1):1–10.

Transesophageal echocardiography

Salim Baghdadi[1] and Balendu C. Vasavada[2]

[1] Department of Cardiology, Long Island College Hospital, New York, NY, USA
[2] University Hospital of Brooklyn, Long Island College Hospital, SUNY Downstate Medical Center, New York, NY, USA

CHAPTER 3

Transthoracic echocardiography (TTE) is an essential diagnostic cardiac tool, since it offers superior visualization of posterior cardiac structures because of the close proximity of the esophagus to the posteromedial heart with lack of intervening lung and bone.

Even though transesophageal echocardiography (TEE) is considered a moderately invasive procedure and generally performed with conscious sedation, TEE is safe and major complications such as death, esophageal injury, sustained ventricular tachycardia, and severe angina have been estimated at less than 1 in 5000.

It is extremely important to be aware of the possibility of methemoglobinemia when starting to prepare a patient for a TEE.

- It is a potentially life-threatening complication of topical benzocaine and related agents used for posterior pharyngeal anesthesia.
- It may be suspected clinically by the development of dyspnea and cyanosis in the presence of a normal arterial PO2.
- Pulse oximetry is inaccurate in monitoring oxygen saturation in the presence of methemoglobinemia and cannot be used to make the diagnosis.
- Early symptoms include headache, fatigue, dyspnea, and lethargy. At higher methemoglobin levels, respiratory depression, altered consciousness, shock, seizures, and death may occur.

Treatment of methemoglobinemia

- Asymptomatic patient with methemoglobin level <20% – no therapy is needed.
- If the patient is symptomatic, or if the methemoglobin level is >20% – specific therapy with methylene blue is indicated.

Practical Manual of Echocardiography in the Urgent Setting, First Edition.
Edited by Vladimir Fridman and Mario J. Garcia.
© 2013 John Wiley & Sons, Ltd. Published 2013 by John Wiley & Sons, Ltd.

Box 3.1 Main indications for TEE

- Evaluation of native valve function, not fully discernible on TTE
- Any prosthetic valve malfunction
- Evaluation for LV and left atrial appendage thrombus
- Evaluation of cardiac masses
- Suspicion of endocarditis
- Aortic dissection
- Guidance of specific interventional/surgical procedures (such as percutaneous ASD repair).

- Methylene blue is given intravenously in a dose of 1–2 mg/kg over five minutes.
- Blood transfusion or exchange transfusion may be helpful in patients who are in shock.
- The response to methylene blue is usually rapid; the dose may be repeated in one hour if the level of methemoglobin is still high.

The 2011 ACCF/ASE/AHA/ASNC/HFSA/HRS/SCAI/SCCM/SCCT/ SCMR 2011 Appropriateness Use Criteria for Echocardiography list appropriate, uncertain, and inappropriate reasons for the use of echocardiography (Box 3.1) [1].

Preparation of the patient

1 Make sure no contraindications to TEE exist (Box 3.2).
2 Patient should be without food and drink for at least four hours prior to the procedure.
3 TEE procedure should be explained in detail to the patient, including the benefits, the risks; and the alternative to the TEE. Consent should be obtained.

Box 3.2 Contraindications to TEE

- Esophageal stricture or malignancy
- Surgical interposition of the esophagus
- Recent esophageal ulcer or hemorrhage
- Zenker's diverticulum
- Altered mental status or an uncooperative patient
- History of odynophagia or dysphagia (need screening endoscopy and/or barium swallow prior to TEE).

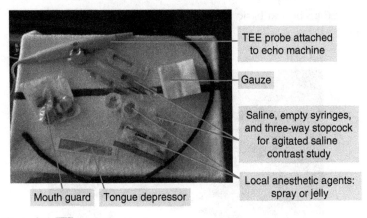

Figure 3.1 TEE set-up.

Box 3.3 Major steps involved in preparing the environment for TEE

1 All proper personnel should be in place and all pre-procedure protocols (such as time out) should be performed.
2 Place patient in the left lateral decubitus position.
3 Artificial teeth/dentures are removed.
4 All local/moderate anesthesia is given to patient.
5 Patient's head is placed in the flexed position and mouth guard is applied.

---

4 A 20 gauge IV should be placed in the patient for administration of medication and contrast agents.
5 Lidocaine hydrochloride spray (or gel) is used for topical anesthesia, which should cover the posterior pharynx and the tongue.
6 Tongue depressor can be used to stimulate gag reflex and the absence of gag reflex means adequate topical anesthesia.
7 Moderate sedation can be used as per hospital protocol. Careful monitoring of the patient's blood pressure, heart rate, and oxygen saturation should be performed during and immediately after the procedure.
8 For contact precaution/special precaution patients-specific contact precaution protocols must be followed regarding probe handling. Please refer to your echo lab manuals for specific protocols.

Appropriate pre-TEE set-up is shown in Figure 3.1 and the steps involved in patient positioning are shown in Box 3.3.

The TEE probe and basic manipulation during the study are shown in Figure 3.2.

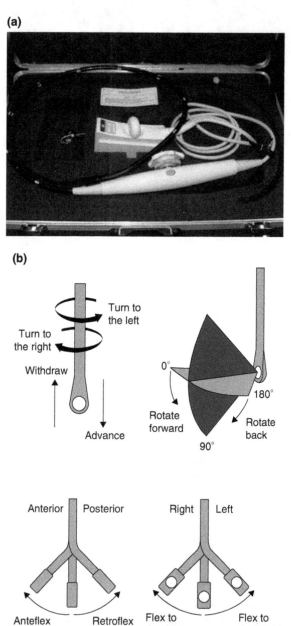

(a)

(b)

Turn to the left

Turn to the right

Withdraw

Advance

0°

Rotate forward

90°

180°

Rotate back

Anterior   Posterior

Anteflex   Retroflex

Right   Left

Flex to the right   Flex to the left

Figure 3.2 **(a)** TEE probe and **(b)** basic manipulation of the probe during TEE (Reproduced from Shanewise *et al.* [2], with permission from Elsevier).

Acoustic windows and standard views

Just like in TTE, there is no required sequence of views for performing a TEE. However, the most frequently used sequence of acquisition is presented here. The operator must remember, nevertheless, that cardiac anatomy may vary according to the patient position and body habitus and underlying cardiac disease. Therefore, quite often, additional probe manipulations may be required to optimize each view.

- Transgastric (TG) mid short axis (SAX) view (Figure 3.3)
  1 Insert the probe to the stomach, probe tip depth 40–45 cm, angle 0–10°.
  2 Advance probe until the stomach (rugae) or liver is seen.
  3 Anteflex to contact stomach wall and inferior wall of heart.
  4 Center left ventricle (LV) by turning probe right or left.
  5 Both papillary muscles imaged.
  6 Increase the gain and lower frequency to optimize endocardial definition.
  7 In the TG mid-SAX view the imaging plane is directed transversely through the mid inferior wall of the LV with all six mid-LV segments viewed at once from the stomach.
- Transgastric basal short axis view (Figure 3.4)
  1 From TG mid-SAX view, withdraw the probe until the mitral valve (MV) is seen in SAX.
  2 Aim to see symmetric MV commissures.
  3 This permits a view of the MV that is parallel to the annulus with the posterior segments of the anterior (A3) and posterior (P3) leaflets and the posterior commissure closest to the probe. This also allows the echocardiographer to determine the mitral valve area via planimetry.

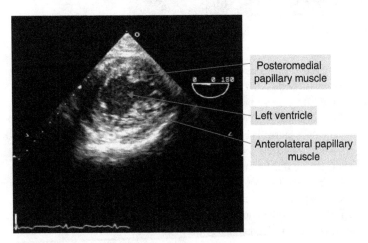

Figure 3.3 Transgastric mid short axis view.

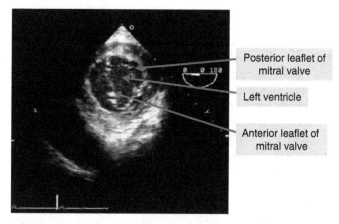

Figure 3.4 Transgastric basal short axis view.

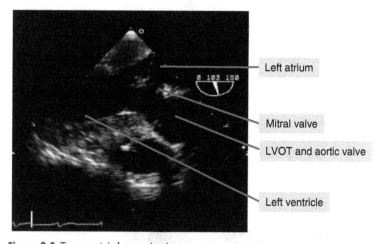

Figure 3.5 Transgastric long axis view.

- Transgastric long axis (LAX) view (Figure 3.5)
  1 From TG two-chamber (90°) view, rotate omniplane angle to 110–120°.
  2 May turn probe to right.
  3 The aortic valve (AV) is seen on the right side of display, adjust depth.
  4 This view permits better spectral Doppler alignment for AV and left ventricle outflow tract (LVOT).
- Transgastric right ventricular inflow (Figure 3.6)
  1 From mid-TG SAX (0°) view, rotate probe clockwise to place right ventricle (RV) in center.
  2 Rotate omniplane angle to 90–120°.
  3 Anteflex until RV is horizontal.

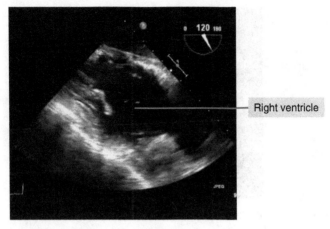

Figure 3.6 Transgastric right ventricular inflow.

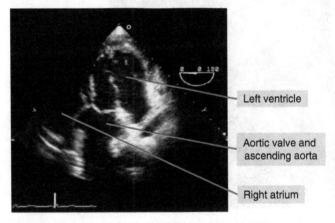

Figure 3.7 Deep transgastric long axis view.

- Deep transgastric long axis view (Figure 3.7)
  1 From mid or apical TG SAX views, anteflex and gently advance probe, hugging the stomach mucosa until the LV apex is seen at the top of the display.
  2 Excessive anteflexion brings image plane superior through base of heart. This image may be used to measure the Doppler derived velocity of flow across the LVOT or AV.
- Mid-esophageal (ME) four-chamber view (Figure 3.8)
  1 Withdraw probe to the mid-esophageal position; probe tip depth 30–40 cm, angle 0–10°.
  2 Image all four heart chambers.

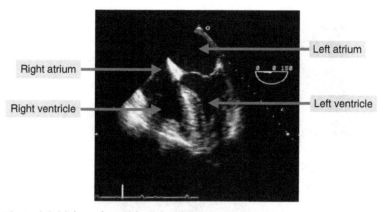

Figure 3.8 Mid-esophageal four-chamber view.

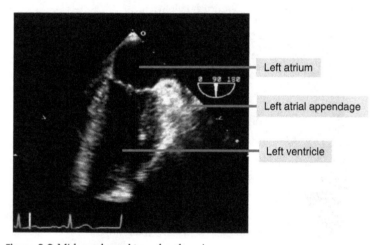

Figure 3.9 Mid-esophageal two-chamber view.

3 Optimize the LV apex by slight retroflexion of probe tip.
4 Ensure no part of the aortic valve or LVOT is seen. Adjust depth to view entire LV, if necessary rotating up to 30°.
- Mid-esophageal two-chamber view (Figure 3.9)
  1 From ME four-chamber (0°) or ME mitral commissural (60°) views, keep the probe tip still and the MV in the center.
  2 Rotate omniplane angle forward to 80–100°.
  3 Right atrium (RA) and right ventricle (RV) disappear, left atrial appendage (LAA appears).
  4 Retroflex probe tip for true LV apex, adjust depth so entire LV apex seen.

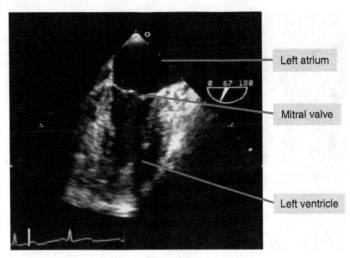

Figure 3.10 Mid-esophageal mitral commissural view.

- Mid-esophageal mitral commissural view (Figure 3.10)
  1 Find the mid-esophageal four-chamber (0°) view.
  2 Keep the probe tip still and the MV in the center.
  3 Rotate omniplane angle forward to 45–60°.
  4 Watch RA and RV disappear.
  5 Retroflex slightly for LV apex.
- Mid-esophageal long axis view (Figure 3.11)
  1 From mid-esophageal two-chamber (90°) view, keep the probe tip still and the MV in the center.
  2 Rotate omniplane angle forward to 120–130°.
  3 AV and LVOT visualized in LAX.
  4 Depth adjusted to keep all of LV in view.
- Mid-esophageal aortic valve long axis view (Figure 3.12)
  1 Find mid-esophageal LAX (120°) view; decrease depth to focus on aortic root.
  2 This view can also be obtained from the mid-esophageal AV SAX (30–60°) view by rotate omniplane angle to 120–150°.
  3 LVOT, AV, proximal ascending aorta line up.
  4 Optimize aortic annulus and make the sinuses of Valsalva symmetric.
- Mid-esophageal aortic valve short axis view (Figure 3.13)
  1 Find the mid-esophageal four-chamber (0°) view, withdraw cephalad to obtain the mid-esophageal five-chamber (0°) view that includes the LVOT and AV.
  2 Rotate omniplane angle to 30–45°.

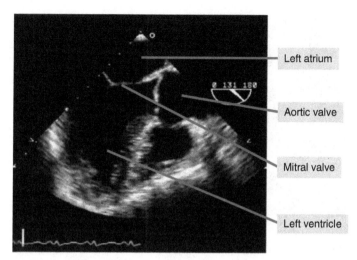

Figure 3.11 Mid-esophageal long axis view.

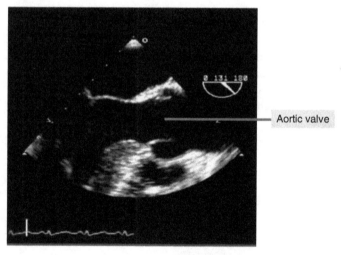

Figure 3.12 Mid-esophageal aortic valve long axis view.

3 Center aortic valve and aim to make three aortic valve cusps symmetric.

4 Withdraw probe for coronary ostia.

5 Advance probe for LVOT.

- Mid-esophageal right ventricular inflow-outflow view (Figure 3.14)
  1 From the mid-esophageal AV SAX (30–60°) view, rotate the omniplane angle to 60–75°.
  2 Optimize tricuspid valve leaflets, open up right ventricle outflow tract (RVOT), bring pulmonary vein and main pulmonary artery into view.

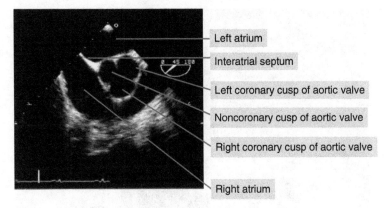

Figure 3.13 Mid-esophageal aortic valve short axis view.

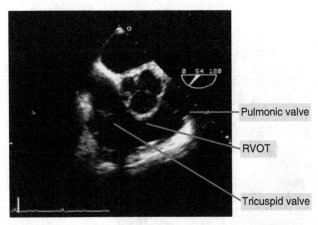

Figure 3.14 Mid-esophageal right ventricular inflow-outflow view.

- Mid-esophageal bicaval view (Figure 3.15)
  1 Find the mid-esophageal two-chamber (90°) view, turn the entire probe right.
  2 Change angle or rotate probe slightly to image both the inferior vena cava (IVC) (left) and superior vena cava (SVC) (right) simultaneously.
- Descending aorta short axis view (Figure 3.16)
  1 From the mid-esophageal view, angle 0°, turn probe to left to find the aorta.
  2 Place aorta in middle of display.
  3 Decrease depth to 5 cm.
  4 Advance and withdraw probe.

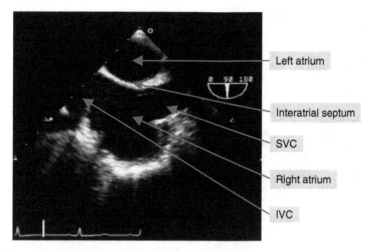

Figure 3.15 Mid-esophageal bicaval view.

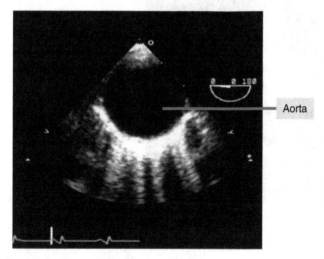

Figure 3.16 Descending aorta short axis view.

- Descending aorta long axis view (Figure 3.17)
  1 From the descending aorta SAX (0°) view, keep probe tip still, rotate omniplane angle to 90–100°.
  2 Aortic walls appear in parallel.
- Upper esophageal aortic arch long axis view (Figure 3.18)
  1 From mid-esophageal descending aorta SAX (0°) view.
  2 Withdraw probe until aorta changes into oval shape; probe tip 20–25 cm, angle 0°.
  3 Turn probe slightly to the right.

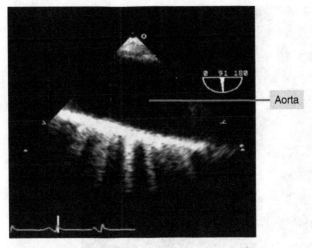

Figure 3.17 Descending aorta long axis view.

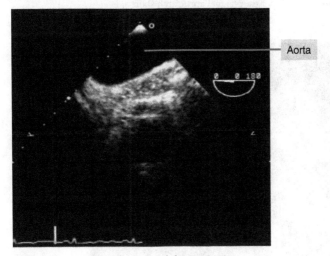

Figure 3.18 Upper esophageal aortic arch long axis view.

- Upper esophageal aortic arch short axis view (Figure 3.19)
  1 From upper-esophageal aortic arch LAX (0°) view, rotate the omniplane angle to 60–90°.
  2 Bring the pulmonic valve and pulmonary artery in view.
- Mid-esophageal ascending aortic short axis view (Figure 3.20)
  1 From mid-esophageal AV LAX (120°) view, withdraw probe (ascending aorta LAX), rotate the omniplane angle back to 0°.

In summary, 20 specific TEE views as recommended in a routine comprehensive TEE examination are shown in Figure 3.21.

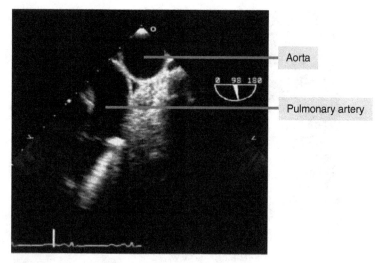

Figure 3.19 Upper esophageal aortic arch short axis view.

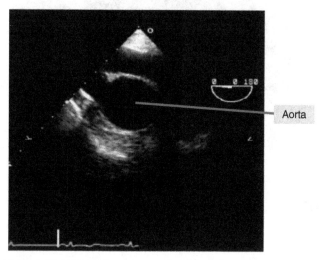

Figure 3.20 Mid-esophageal ascending aortic short axis view.

Clean-up and maintenance

• Probes should be rinsed with warm water immediately. The rinse should be one minute and a large volume of fresh water should be used.

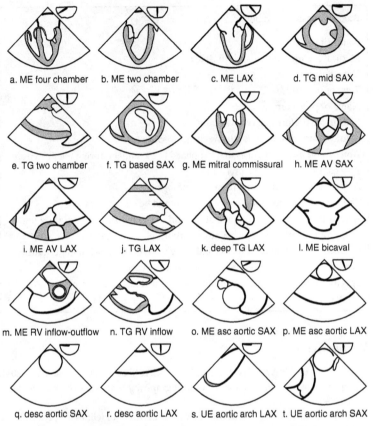

a. ME four chamber   b. ME two chamber   c. ME LAX   d. TG mid SAX

e. TG two chamber   f. TG based SAX   g. ME mitral commissural   h. ME AV SAX

i. ME AV LAX   j. TG LAX   k. deep TG LAX   l. ME bicaval

m. ME RV inflow-outflow   n. TG RV inflow   o. ME asc aortic SAX   p. ME asc aortic LAX

q. desc aortic SAX   r. desc aortic LAX   s. UE aortic arch LAX   t. UE aortic arch SAX

Figure 3.21 Twenty TEE views that comprise a comprehensive TEE examination (Reproduced from Shanewise *et al.* [2], with permission from Elsevier).

Dry the probe with a paper towel and make sure no secretions are left on the probe after the rinse.

• As for preparing TEE probes, probes that come from patients with contact precautions/special precautions should be cleaned as per the special laboratory protocols for those types of patients.

• Probes should be cleaned in high level disinfection as per the echo laboratory protocol.

After the TEE is performed, a preliminary report should be placed in the chart, and a full report should follow as soon as possible. Important parts of preliminary and final reports are listed in Box 3.4.

Box 3.4 Basic TEE report

Name of patient
Medical record number and/or date of birth
Date of procedure
Time of procedure
Name of procedure
Reason for performing of procedure
Medications administered during the procedure
Any hemodynamic changes that happened to the patient during the procedure
Any complications of the procedure
Any pertinent positive and negative findings
The clinical question for the procedure should be clearly answered.
An impression should be made at the end of the report clearly stating the
appropriate positive and negative findings of the procedure.
Detailed description of cardiac chambers, valves, great vessels and pericardium
Results of any calculations or quantitative measurements
Specific post-procedure recommendations, such as maintaining of NPO
status.

References

1 ACCF/ASE/AHA/ASNC/HFSA/HRS/SCAI/SCCM/SCCT/SCMR 2011 Appropriate use criteria for echocardiography. *J Am Soc Echocardiogr* 2011; 24:229–67.
2 Shanewise JS, Cheung AT, Aronson S, *et al.* ASE/SCA Guidelines for performing a comprehensive intraoperative multiplane transesophageal echocardiography examination: Recommendations of the American Society of Echocardiography Council for Intraoperative Echocardiography and the Society of Cardiovascular Anesthesiologists Task Force for Certification in Perioperative Transesophageal Echocardiography. *J Am Soc Echocardiogr* 1999; 12:884–900.

Ventricles

Deepika Misra[1] and Dayana Eslava[2]

[1] Beth Israel Medical Center, New York, NY, USA
[2] St Luke's Roosevelt Hospital, New York, NY, USA

CHAPTER 4

Left ventricle

The left ventricle (LV) is the most important chamber to examine in the critically ill patient. The echocardiographic examination of the left ventricle should include assessment of chamber size, mass, functional assessment, diastolic dysfunction, and regional wall motion.

Chamber size

Measurements of LV size may be obtained by M-mode, 2D or 3D imaging. In the critically ill patient, 2D derived measurements are often the most reliable. When obtained, M-mode tracings should be obtained in the parasternal long axis view as perpendicular to the LV cavity as possible at the tips of the mitral leaflets (Figure 4.1a). A short axis view may be used as well.

- The end diastolic diameter (LVIDd) is measured at the maximum separation of the septum and posterior wall, at the onset of the QRS complex from leading edge to leading edge [1].
- The end systolic dimension (LVIDs) is measured at the peak downward motion of the septal wall. Septal and posterior wall thickness is measured at the onset of the QRS. Normal measurements for these dimensions are shown in Tables 4.1 and 4.2.

Using M-mode imaging of the LV, fractional shortening (FS) – a measure of LV contractility – can be obtained using the formula:

$$FS(\%) = (LVIDd - LVIDs) / LVIDd \times 100$$

The normal FS is 25–45%.

Using 2D imaging, apical views are excellent for providing the necessary components to measure left ventricular size and function.

Practical Manual of Echocardiography in the Urgent Setting, First Edition.
Edited by Vladimir Fridman and Mario J. Garcia.
© 2013 John Wiley & Sons, Ltd. Published 2013 by John Wiley & Sons, Ltd.

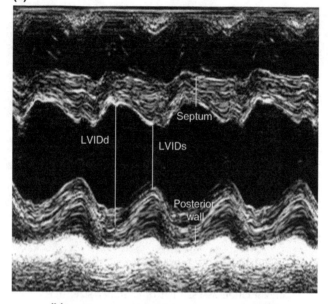

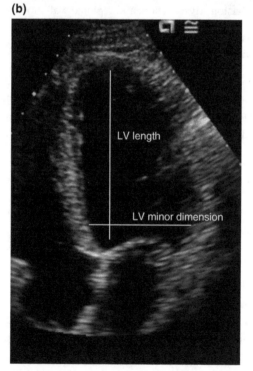

Figure 4.1 M-mode **(a)** and apical four-chamber **(b)** views of the left ventricle. Many of the necessary LV dimensions (cavity size, wall thickness, ejection fraction) can be derived from these views.

Measurements of the internal LV length and of the LV minor dimension can be made in these views (Figure 4.1b). Measurements by 2D should be done only if good quality images of the LV, without foreshortening and with good endocardial definition, are obtained.

LV volume assessment is performed by two methods, as recommended by the American Society of Echocardiography (ASE):

1 Area–length method:
- LV is assumed to have a bullet shape.
- The area of the LV is measured in the parasternal short axis view by planimetry.
- The length of the ventricle is measured in the apical four-chamber view from the midpoint of the mitral annulus to the apex.
- The volume is calculated by the formula: volume = {5(area)(length)}/6. The volumes are calculated in systole and diastole [2].

2 Biplane Modified Simpson's Method (Figure 4.2):
- Total LV volume is calculated from the summation of elliptical disks.
- The LV is divided into 20 disks.
- The volume of each disk is $\Pi \times a/2 \times b/2 \times h$, where a and b are the disk diameters determined in two apical views and h is the height of each disk [2]. Typically, the length of the long axis of the LV (L) is divided equally into 20 disks, so h=L/20 [2].
- In modern echocardiographic machines, this calculation can be performed automatically.
- To perform the calculation, the endocardial border should be traced in systole (at the point when the LV cavity is the smallest of the systolic period) and in diastole (at the point when the LV cavity is the largest of the diastolic period) (Figure 4.2).

Mass

LV mass is an important factor in the future development of reduced left ventricular function and heart failure.

The principle of LV mass measurement:
- Involves subtraction of the LV cavity volume from the volume of the LV epicardium.
- The resultant volume of the LV muscle is then multiplied by the specific gravity of the myocardium, 1.04 g/ml, to give the LV mass.
- The LV mass can be calculated from M-mode measurements of the LV by the formula proposed by Devereaux *et al.* [3] and is:

$$LV\,mass\,(linear\,method) = 0.8 \times \left\{ 1.04[(LVIDd + PWTd + SWTd)^3 \right.$$

$$\left. - (LVIDd)^3] \right\} + 0.6g$$

(LVIDd is the LV internal diameter in diastole, PWT is posterior wall thickness at end diastole, SWTd is septal wall thickness at end diastole).

Table 4.1 Normal chamber quantification measurements.

	Women				Men			
	Ref Range	Mildly abnormal	Mod abnormal	Severely abnormal	Ref Range	Mild abnormal	Mod abnormal	Severely abnormal
LA diameter, cm	2.7–3.8	3.9–4.2	4.3–4.6	≥4.7	3.0–4.0	4.1–4.6	4.7–5.2	≥5.2
LA diameter/BSA, cm/m²	1.5–2.3	2.4–2.6	2.7–2.9	≥3.0	1.5–2.3	2.4–2.6	2.7–2.9	≥3.0
RA minor-axis dimension, cm	2.9–4.5	4.6–4.9	5.0–5.4	≥5.5	2.9–4.5	4.6–4.9	5.0–5.4	≥5.5
LA minor axis dimension/BSA, cm/m²	1.7–2.5	2.6–2.8	2.9–3.1	≥3.2	1.7–2.5	2.6–2.8	2.9–3.1	≥3.2
LA area, cm²	≤20	20–30	30–40	>40	≤20	20–30	30–40	>40
LA volume, ml	22–52	53–62	63–72	≥73	18–58	59–68	69–78	≥79
LA volume/BSA, ml/m²	22±6	29–33	34–39	≥40	22±6	29–33	34–39	≥40
LV diastolic diameter, cm	3.9–5.3	5.4–5.7	5.8–6.1	≥6.2	4.2–5.9	6.0–6.3	6.4–6.8	≥6.9
LV diastolic diameter/BSA, cm/m²	2.4–3.2	3.3–3.4	3.5–3.7	≥3.8	2.2–3.1	3.2–3.4	3.5–3.6	≥3.8
LV diastolic volume, ml	56–104	105–117	118–130	≥131	67–155	156–178	179–201	≥201
LV diastolic volume/BSA, ml/m²	35–75	76–86	87–96	≥97	35–75	76–86	87–96	≥97
LV systolic volume, ml	19–49	50–59	60–69	≥70	22–58	59–70	71–82	≥83
LV systolic volume/BSA, ml/m²	12–30	31–36	37–42	≥43	12–30	31–36	37–42	≥43

LV function

	Ref Range	Mild abnormal	Mod abnormal	Severely abnormal				
Endocardial fractional shortening, %	27–45	22–26	17–21	≤16	25–43	20–24	15–19	≤14
2D Ejection fraction, %	≥55	45–54	30–44	<30	≥55	45–54	30–44	<30

LV mass

	Ref Range	Mild abnormal	Mod abnormal	Severely abnormal				
LV mass, g	67–162	163–186	187–210	≥211	88–224	225–258	259–292	≥293
LV mass/BSA, g/m²	43–95	96–108	109–121	≥122	49–115	116–131	132–148	≥149
Septal thickness, cm	0.6–0.9	1.0–1.2	1.3–1.5	≥1.6	0.6–1.0	1.1–1.3	1.4–1.6	≥1.7
Posterior wall thickness, cm	0.6–0.9	1.0–1.2	1.3–1.5	≥1.6	0.6–1.0	1.1–1.3	1.4–1.6	≥1.7

RV dimensions

	Ref Range	Mild abnormal	Mod abnormal	Severely abnormal
Basal RV diameter (level of tricuspid valve), cm	2.0–2.8	2.9–3.3	3.4–3.8	≥3.9
Mid-RV diameter, cm	2.7–3.3	3.4–3.7	3.8–4.1	≥4.2
Base-to-apex length, cm	7.1–7.9	8.0–8.5	8.6–9.1	≥9.2
RV diastolic area, cm²	11–28	29–32	33–37	≥38
RV systolic area, cm²	7.5–16	17–19	20–22	≥23
RV fractional area change, %	32–60	25–31	18–24	≤17

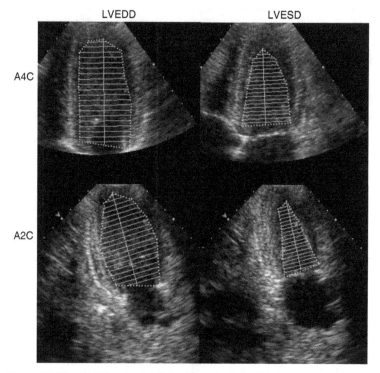

Figure 4.2 Modified Simpson's Method for calculating LV volumes using the apical four-chamber (A4C) and apical two-chamber (A2C) views.

LV mass using the 2D method is calculated based on the area–length method and the truncated ellipsoid formula. For the purpose of this book detailed information on calculation by 2D methods is not provided.

Once LV mass is calculated, if an increased LV mass is noted, further investigation is warranted. It is extremely important to note that LV mass can be increased without the presence of left ventricular hypertrophy (LVH) on ECG. Relative wall thickness (RWT) permits categorization of an increase in LV mass as either concentric or eccentric (Figure 4.3).

$$RWT = (2 \times PWTd) / LVIDd$$

RWT >/= 0.42 is consistent with concentric hypertrophy, RWT </= 0.42 is consistent with eccentric hypertrophy [4].

Functional assessment
In any emergent clinical situation, the most critical part of LV assessment is its functional status. Treatment usually is based on the results of this

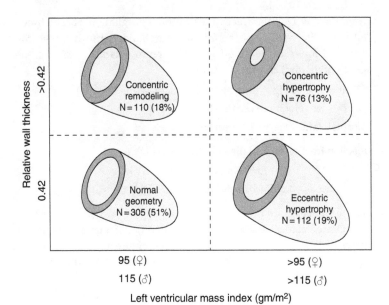

Figure 4.3 Three types of left ventricular hypertrophy, as defined by the VALIANT trial [5, 6].

assessment, and thus it is extremely important that a thorough and accurate assessment is performed.

LV systolic function can be measured using multiple techniques:

- Visual estimation – depends on reader experience but has considerable inter-observer variability.
- Fractional shortening/Ejection fraction measured by M-mode is an indicator of systolic function. However, if there is any wall motion abnormality, it is inaccurate.
- Doppler assessment of LV stroke volume. Stroke volume (SV) is the volume of blood ejected by the left ventricle with each systole

Stroke volume = VTI of LVOT × Area of LVOT

To perform this calculation, first measure the LVOT diameter (radius = ½ diameter). Πr^2 is the area of the LVOT. VTI is the velocity time integral of the all the velocities within the Doppler spectrum of flow obtained from the LVOT. It is obtained by tracing the PW Doppler signal taken at the LVOT in systole. The flow and diameter measurements must be done at the same site for accurate determination of SV [7]. For the calculation of cardiac output, the formula: Cardiac Output = SV × heart rate is used.

- Doppler dP/dt as a measure of contractility: dP/dt is the rate of LV pressure change during isovolumic contraction. It can be measured from the CW Doppler trace of the mitral regurgitation jet. The time it takes for the velocity of the mitral regurgitation jet to increase from 1 m/s to 3 m/s is measured (dt). This represents a LV–LA pressure gradient dP ($4v^2$) change of 32 mm Hg.

$$dP/dt = 32 \text{ mm Hg} / \text{(time needed to increase the MR jet velocity in seconds)}$$

Normal values are > 1200 mm Hg/s.

$$\text{Ejection fraction} = \big(\text{End diastolic volume}(\text{EDV})\big)$$
$$-\text{End systolic volume }(\text{ESV})\big) /$$
$$\text{End diastolic volume }(\text{EDV}).$$

The normal ejection fraction by this method is >/=55%.

Volumes are calculated using the modified Simpson method as described in the LV quantification section (Figure 4.2). The apex must not be foreshortened for these calculations and two orthogonal views are required [2].

- New methods: LV function can be assessed by using global or regional strain or strain rate. Also, 3D echo provides better volume measurements than 2D echo for assessment of LV function [2].

Diastolic dysfunction

Diastole starts at aortic valve closure and includes rapid filling of the left ventricle in early diastole followed by a period of diastasis and then atrial contraction. Abnormalities of diastolic function can lead to severe heart failure symptoms, irrespective of the patient's systolic function.

Several indicators on echocardiography are measured to assess diastolic dysfunction. The following parameters are indicators of diastolic dysfunction:

- Increased left atrium (LA) volume: As filling pressures are high in the LV over a period of time, the left atrium dilates to accommodate for the increased left ventricular filling pressures.
- Abnormal LV filling pulsed Doppler (Figure 4.4): This measures the gradient between the LA and the LV in diastole. The E wave represents peak velocity during rapid filling and the A wave represents peak velocity after atrial contraction. The deceleration time (DT) represents the operating compliance of the LV and is traced from the peak of the E wave to the baseline.
- In normal diastolic filling, the E wave is greater than the A wave and DT is between 160 and 240 msec (Figure 4.5).
- Abnormal mitral annular velocities: Tissue Doppler imaging is recorded from the medial and lateral aspects of the mitral annulus in the apical four-chamber view. The e′ and a′ velocities are recorded (Figure 4.6). The E/e′ ratio is an indicator of LV filling pressures

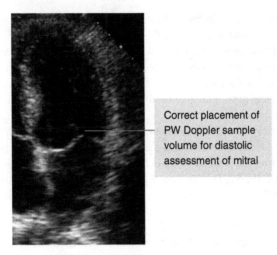

Correct placement of PW Doppler sample volume for diastolic assessment of mitral

Figure 4.4 Abnormal LV filling pulsed Doppler.

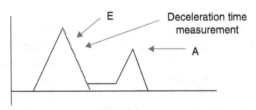

Figure 4.5 E and A velocities, and deceleration time measurement (dashed red line) of mitral valve inflow.

(cannot be used in normal subjects/heavy annular calcification/mitral valve disease/constrictive pericarditis). A ratio <8 represents normal filling pressure and ratio >15 determines elevated filling pressures [8, 9]. A ratio between 8 and 15 is inconclusive.

- Diastolic dysfunction grading (Table 4.2, Figure 4.6):
  ○ Grade I – As diastolic dysfunction progresses, the A wave velocity increases such that the E/A ratio is reversed and the DT is prolonged.
  ○ Grade II (Pseudonormal pattern) – occurs as the LA pressure increases with worsening diastolic dysfunction and the E/A ratio returns to normal. It can differentiated from the normal pattern by the use of tissue Doppler (E' <8cm/s, E/E' >15)
  ○ Grade III – characterized by the E/A ratio increasing and the DT shortening; this is a poor prognostic indicator.
  ○ Grade IV – same as grade III if persisting after use of diuretics or Valsalva.

Of note, a decrease in the E/A ratio by 50% with the Valsalva maneuver also is an indicator of increased LVEDP [8, 9].

It is important to note that it is difficult in some echocardiogram machines to switch to the Doppler Tissue Interface (DTI) mode, which is required for recording of mitral annular velocities. Please read the instructions, and make sure the correct mode is chosen, prior to acquisition.

- Pulmonary vein flow velocities: There are two systolic velocities, S1 (atrial relaxation) and S2, and a diastolic velocity (D). As LV relaxation is impaired the ratio of S2 to D increases. Conversely, as LA pressure increases, the S2/D ratio decreases. The duration of the retrograde A wave in the pulmonary veins increase as LVEDP rises. A pulmonary A wave duration – LV inflow A wave duration >30 msec is associated with increased LVEDP [10, 11].

Normal and abnormal diastolic function measurements are shown in Table 4.2 and Figure 4.6.

Regional wall motion assessment

The ASE has divided the ventricle into 16 segments for purposes of wall motion analysis in 1989. The American Heart Association (AHA) has recommended a 17-segment model to make echo studies comparable to myocardial perfusion studies.

In the 16-segment model, the LV is divided into apical, mid and basal levels. The basal and mid-level are divided into the anteroseptum, anterior, anterolateral, inferolateral, inferior and inferoseptum. The apical segment consists of the septum, anterior, lateral and inferior segments [13, 14] The 17-segment model adds the apical cap (which is beyond the LV cavity) and is used for myocardial perfusion studies [15]. This model is shown in Chapter 2.

Wall motion is scored according to the following:

1 = Normal/hyperkinetic
2 = Hypokinetic
3 = Akinetic
4 = Dyskinetic
5 = Aneurysmal

Right ventricle

Echocardiographic evaluation of the right ventricle (RV) can be difficult due to its crescent shape and irregular or trabeculated endocardial surface (caused by muscle bundles, particularly the moderator band). However,

Table 4.2 Diastolic function measurements.

	E/A ratio	e' (septal) (cm/s)	E/e'	DT (ms)	AR (ms)	AR dur	PV trace	LA size
Normal	>1.5	>10	<8	140<DT<220	<0.35	<Adur	S≥D	normal
Grade 1	<1.0	<8	<8	>220	<0.35	<Adur	S>D	normal or dilated (>/=34 ml/m²)
Grade 2	1–1.5	<8	>15	140<DT<220	>0.35	> Adur+30msec	S<D	dilated
Grade 3–4	>2	<8	>15	DT <150	>0.35	> Adur+30msec	S<D	dilated

AR – peak atrial reversal flow velocity of pulmonary vein flow; AR dur – duration of AR; Adur – duration of A wave of mitral inflow; DT – deceleration time; PV – pulmonary vein; S – peak systolic PV velocity; D – peak diastolic PV velocity

Note: Some grade 1 diastolic dysfunction patients have elevated LVEDP and E/e'>15.

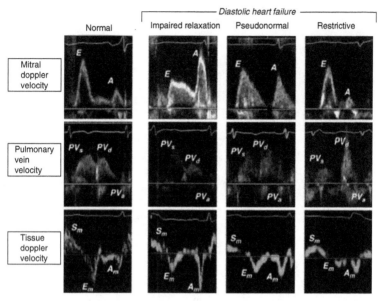

Figure 4.6 Diastolic function assessment, as seen on echocardiography of mitral inflow (top row), pulmonic flow (middle row), and tissue Doppler velocity of mitral valve annulus (bottom row) (Reproduced from Abraham and Abraham [12], with permission from Elsevier).

the most reliable method to identify which chamber is the RV is its association with the tricuspid valve. Like the LV, the RV should be assessed by using multiple windows [16]:

- Parasternal long axis view (PLAX): This view places the RV in near field with both the endocardial and epicardial surfaces nearly perpendicular to the ultrasound beam. This view can be used to estimate the RV size and to evaluate the ventricular septal motion.
- Short axis view: This view can be used to define the papillary muscles and the chordal insertions (which are used to identify the ventricles).
- Apical four-chamber view: This is the best view to determine ventricular morphology and the relative positions of the atrioventricular valves as well as the integrity of the valves. This view can also be used to estimate the RV size by comparing its size relative to that of the LV:
  - RV < LV = Normal
  - RV = LV = mildly-to-moderately enlarged
  - RV > LV = severely enlarged.
  - Normally the RV size is approximately two-thirds that of the LV.

- Subcostal four-chamber view: This view provides the best visualization of the RV free wall and provides the most reliable estimate of RV size and RV systolic function. It is also ideal (along with the short axis view) for assessing the complex geometry and for determining the level and severity of the tricuspid valve stenosis.

The echocardiographic characteristics of the RV are:
- Trabeculated endocardial surface.
- Three papillary muscles.
- Chordae insert into the ventricular septum.
- Infundibular muscle band.
- Moderator band.
- Triangular cavity shape.
- Tricuspid atrioventricular valve with relatively apical insertion.

Measuring RV volume

- Area–length method: requires two measurements, an estimate of short axis and a linear measure of length (from the apical four-chamber view, as seen in Figure 4.7). (Reference values are shown in Table 4.1.).
- The RV is also measured using planimetry from the four-chamber view.

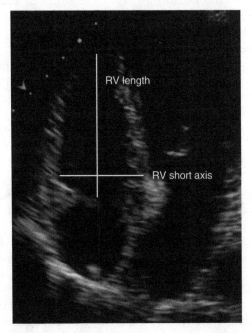

Figure 4.7 Apical four-chamber view.

- 3D Echo: Renders a more precise view of the RV cavity and eliminates assumptions about the shape of the RV.

Evaluation of RV systolic function [2, 16]

- Qualitative assessment of the RV contractility can be made from multiple views. However, the best views are the apical four-chamber and the subcostal view (most reliable view). The RV systolic function can be graded in comparison with the LV systolic function. Regional or global wall motion can be graded for the extent and severity of dysfunction as normal, mildly, moderately, or severely reduced. The free wall and interventricular septum should be evaluated for thickening and endocardial excursion.
- Quantitative assessment can be carried out by:
  - ○ Tricuspid annular plane systolic excursion (TAPSE –the distance the tricuspid annulus moves in the antero–posterior direction). This can be evaluated with M-mode, 2D echo, or tissue Doppler in the apical four-chamber view. This method has greater reproducibility.
  - ○ Tricuspid fractional shortening (assessment of the difference between the maximal and the minimal distance between the tricuspid annuli during the cardiac cycle).
  - ○ RV fractional area change (RVFAC): this can be determined by measuring the RV areas, in the apical four-chamber view, and comparing the relative change between diastole and systole. This method correlates best with MRI.

The RV is able to eject a large volume of blood, with minimal degree of myocardial shortening, due to the low pulmonary vascular resistance. Consequently, an abnormal RV wall motion can occur in patients with pulmonary hypertension and/or pulmonary embolus. RV dysfunction can also occur in conditions such as inferior myocardial dysfunction and arrhythmogenic RV dysplasia. This is discussed in later chapters.

Determination of the central venous pressure (Table 4.3)

- The junction of the inferior vena cava (IVC) and the right atrium (RA) is visualized from the subcostal view.
- The IVC diameter is measured and used to estimate the RA pressure.
- The IVC diameter changes with changes in the central venous pressure (CVP) and the respiratory cycle, so the degree of IVC collapsibility with inspiration should be assessed.
- Normally the IVC diameter decreases more than 50% during sniffing or inspiration. Therefore, absence of this response suggests an increase in RA pressure.

Table 4.3 Estimation of right atrial pressure.

IVC	Change with Respiration or "Sniff"	Estimated RA pressure, mm Hg
Small (<1.5 cm)	Collapse	0–5
Normal (1.5–2.5 cm)	Decrease by >50%	5–10
	Decrease by <50%	10–15
Dilated (>2.5 cm)	Decrease by <50%	15–20
Dilated with dilated hepatic veins	No change	>20

Estimation of RA pressure from the respiratory variation in the IVC is only useful in spontaneously breathing patients. IVC does not predict RA pressures in patients on mechanical ventilation. IVC measurements with mechanical ventilation are less reliable because of the difference in intra-thoracic pressures with positive pressure ventilation versus normal negative pressure ventilation. In ventilated patients, a measured central venous pressure is used.

Abnormal septal motion in RV volume and/or pressure overload

In the normal heart, the round shape of the LV is maintained throughout the cardiac cycle due to the higher pressure within the LV cavity. However, when the RV pressure increases, the normal septal curvature flattens and is displaced towards the LV such that the LV assumes a D-shape seen in the short axis view. With RV pressure overload, the interventricular septal flattening persists throughout both systole and diastole; in contrary to RV volume overload, where the septal flattening is seen only during diastole. Pressure overload of the RV results in hypertrophy which is associated with an increase in the trabeculations of the RV walls. This is discussed further in later chapters.

Determination of RV systolic pressure

Using the Bernoulli equation, a noninvasive calculation of the RV and PA systolic pressures is possible by quantifying the TR jet velocity. The maximum TR jet velocity measures the RV to RA systolic pressure gradient. The RV systolic pressure=$4\times$(TR jet velocity)^2+RA pressure (estimated using the IVC diameter and its respiratory variation, discussed previously). In the absence of pulmonic stenosis, the RV and PA systolic pressures are

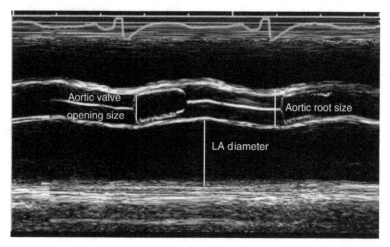

Figure 4.8 The dimensions of the LA can be determined at end-systole in the PLAX view. This is usually done in M-mode.

the same, which provides a simple way to quantify the presence of pulmonary hypertension. When pulmonic stenosis is present, pulmonary systolic pressure is calculated by subtracting the RV to PA gradient from the estimated RV systolic pressure. This is discussed in later chapters.

Atria

Left atrium
- The dimension of the LA can be determined at end-systole in the PLAX view. This is usually done in M-mode (Figure 4.8). However, it may be underestimated from this view because the LA may enlarge longitudinally.

  Therefore, LA size should be measured from the apical views (from the tip of the MV to the posterior wall of the LA).
- LA volume is a better measure of LA size. LA size or volume is an important determinant of LA pressure, diastolic function, and prognosis. Normal and abnormal values of LA size and volume are shown in Table 4.1.

Four different methods are available for determining LA volume:

1 Prolate ellipse method: LA dimensions are measured from the PLAX view and apical four-chamber view.

2 Biplane area–length method (Figure 4.9): measures the LA area from two orthogonal apical views (A1 and A2) and LA length (L), from which LA volume is calculated as $0.85 \times A1 \times A2 / L$. When LA length is measured from two apical views (L1 and L2), the shorter value is used

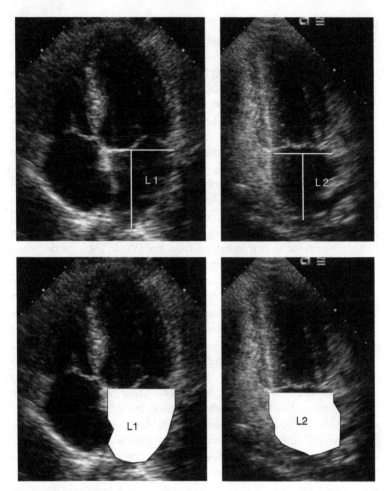

Figure 4.9 Biplane area–length method.

to calculate LA volume. For the area (A) and length (L) measurements in this method, the mitral valve annulus (not leaflet tips) is used as the limit of the left atrium. This method is the one recommended by the American Society of Echocardiography [2].

3 Biplane Simpson – same steps involved as calculating LV volume by this method.

4 3D Echo.

The influence of body surface area on LA volume is corrected by dividing LA volume by body surface area to calculate the LA volume index. The normal value for all age groups for the LA volume index is $22 \pm 6\,\text{ml/m}^2$ [2].

Right atrium

- The RA is a thin walled chamber that can be visualized in several views.
- Its measurements, including planimetry, are usually performed from the apical four-chamber or subcostal view.
- RA size has not been as well studied as the other chambers. For clinical basis, visual comparison of LA and RA size is performed from the apical four-chamber view [2].
- A RA that appears larger than the LA is qualitative evidence of an enlarged chamber.

The RA contains several distinct normal variants, which are occasionally mistaken for pathologic structures. These include the Eustachian valve, Chiari network and crista terminalis (Figures 4.10 and 4.11). The Eustachian valve and Chiari network consists of thin filamentous structures that extend from the IVC to the superior vena cava (SVC) and on imaging appear as bright echoes in the RA. These structures are embryologic remnants that can be visualized from the parasternal right ventricular inflow and subcostal views, though better seen on transesophageal echocardiogram. The Eustachian valve is a protuberant structure (variable sizes), usually immobile that directs the blood from the IVC across the atrial septum to the LA. Failure of this embryologic structure to regress can either be inconsequential or can result in partial or complete septation of the RA, referred to as cor triatriatum dexter. The Chiari network is a more delicate and mobile structure that serves as the valve of the coronary sinus. Both the Eustachian valve and Chiari network are of little clinical significance; however they can be mobile within the RA and thus confused with tumors, vegetations, or thrombi. The crista terminalis, a normal anatomical structure, is a fibromuscular ridge often seen in the transthoracic apical four chamber view as a slight bump on the superior aspect of the RA wall (Figure 4.11).

It is important to recognize these structures as normal variants, and not as abnormal structures.

Contrast echocardiography

If the echocardiographic pictures are suboptimal for any reason, the use of contrast can be utilized. These are specifically based on "microbubbles" that when they receive ultrasound waves can create a strong signal due to the principle of harmonics. Figures 4.12 and 4.13 show a LV prior to and after administration of contrast. Post administration, the LV cavity is much more easily visible and can be analyzed much more accurately. There are multiple contrast agents available commercially. Individual

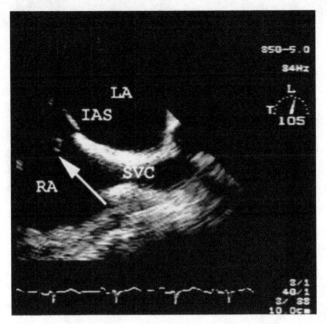

Figure 4.10 Transthoracic echocardiography (TTE) view of eustachian valve in the right atrium (Reproduced from Kerut *et al.* [17], with permission from Elsevier).

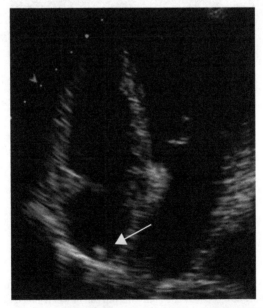

Figure 4.11 Prominenet Crista Terminalis (arrow) is seen in the right atrium. This should not be confused with thrombus of the right atrium.

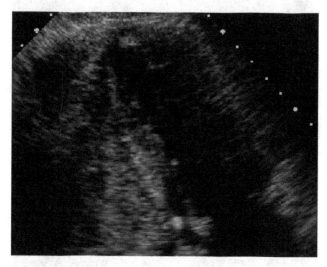

Figure 4.12 The LV endocardium is not visualized in this apical two-chamber view.

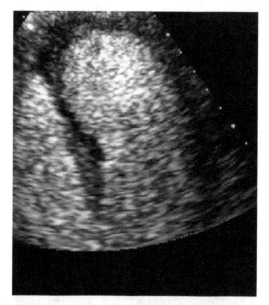

Figure 4.13 The apical view of the LV of the patient in Figure 4.9 after contrast agent has been administered. The endocardium can be easily noted and analyzed in this view.

echocardiography laboratory protocols should be followed for administration of contrast agents.

Overall, chamber quantification is an extremely important part of echocardiography. The sizes of all chambers should be analyzed and extra careful attention should be paid to the RV and LV sizes, due to their importance to patient diagnosis and treatment. Whether normal or abnormal, it is also extremely important to put all the chamber size details in the echocardiography reports and to report them to the medical team treating the patient as soon as possible.

References

1 Feigenbaum H, Armstrong W, Ryan T. *Feigenbaum's Echocardiography*, 6th edn. Philadelphia: Lippincott, Williams and Wilkins, 2005.

2 Lang RM, Bierig M, Devereux RB, *et al*. Recommendations for chamber quantification: A report from the American Society of Echocardiography's guidelines and standard's committee and the chamber quantification group, developed in conjunction with the European Association of Echocardiography, a branch of the European Society of Cardiology. *J Am Soc Echocardiogr* 2005; 18:1440–1463.

3 Devereux RB, Alonso DR, Lutas EM, *et al*. Echocardiographic assessment of left ventricular hypertrophy: comparison to necropsy findings. *Am J Cardiol* 1986; 57:450–8.

4 Ganau A, Devereux RB, Roman MJ, *et al*. Patterns of left ventricular hypertrophy and geometric remodeling in essential hypertension. *J Am Coll Cardiol* 1992; 19:1550–8.

5 Verma A, Meris A, Skali H, *et al*. Prognostic implications of left ventricular mass and geometry following myocardial infarction. *JACC Card Imag* 2008; 1(5):582–91.

6 Konstam MA, Kramer DG, Patel AR, *et al*. Left ventricular remodeling in heart failure: current concepts in clinical significance and assessment. *JACC Card Imag* 2011; 4(1):98–108.

7 Otto CM. (ed.) *Textbook of Clinical Echocardiography*, 3rd edn. Philadelphia: Elsevier Saunders, 2004.

8 Sherif FN, Appleton CP, Gillebert TC, *et al*. Recommendations for the evaluation of left ventricular diastolic function by echocardiography. *J Am Soc Echocardiogr* 2009; Feb 2009:107–133.

9 Ommen SR, Nishimura RA, Appleton CP, *et al*. Clinical utility of Doppler echocardiography and tissue Doppler imaging in the estimation of left ventricular filling pressures: a comparative simultaneous Doppler-catheterization study. *Circulation* 2002; 102:1788–94.

10 Djaiani GN, MCreath BJ, Ti LK, *et al*. Mitral flow propagation velocity identifies patients with abnormal diastolic function during coronary artery bypass graft surgery. *Anesth & Analg* 2002; 95(3):524–30.

11 Dini F, Michelassi C, Micheli G, Rovai D. Prognostic value of pulmonary venous flow Doppler signal in left ventricular dysfunction: a contribution of

the difference in duration of pulmonary venous and mitral flow at atrial contraction. *J Am Coll Cardiol* 2000; 36:1295–302.

12 Abraham J, Abraham TP. The role of echocardiography in hemodynamic assessment in heart failure. *Heart Fail Clin* 2009; 5(2):191–208.

13 Schiller NB, Shah PM, Crawford M, *et al.* Recommendations for quantitation of the left ventricle by two-dimensional echocardiography: American Society of Echocardiography committee on standards, subcommittee on quantitation of of two-dimensional echocardiograms. *J Am Soc Echocardiogr* 1989; 2:358–67.

14 Pellika PA, Nagueh SF, Elhendy AA, *et al.* American Society of Echocardiography recommendations for performance, interpretation, and application of stress echocardiography. *J Am Soc Echocardiogr* 2007; 20:1021–41.

15 Cerqueira MD, Weissman NJ, Dilsizian V, *et al.* Standardized myocardial segmentation and nomenclature for tomographic imaging of the heart: a statement for healthcare professionals from the cardiac imaging committee of the council on clinical cardiology of the American Heart Association. *Circulation* 2002; 105:539–42.

16 Rudski LG, Wyman WW, Afilalo J, *et al.* Guidelines for the echocardiographic assessment of the right heart in adults: A report from the American Society of Echocardiography: Endorsed by the European Association of Echocardiography, a registered branch of the European Society of Cardiology, and the Canadian Society of Echocardiography. *J Am Soc Echocardiogr* 2010; 23(7):685–718.

17 Kerut EK, Norfleet WT, Plotnic GD, Giles TD. Patent foramen ovale: A review of associated conditions and the impact of physiological size. *J Am Coll Cardiol* 2001; 38(3):613–23.

Left-sided heart valves

Muhammad M. Chaudhry[1], Ravi Diwan[1], Yili Huang[1], and Furqan H. Tejani[2]

[1] Beth Israel Medical Center, New York, NY, USA
[2] State University of New York, Downstate Medical Center, University Hospital of Brooklyn at Long Island College Hospital, New York, NY, USA

CHAPTER 5

Aortic valve

Aortic stenosis

Aortic stenosis (AS) is the progressive narrowing of the aortic valve that can lead to left ventricular hypertrophy or systolic dysfunction due to pressure overload. Mortality is high if severe stenosis remains untreated.

A triad of symptoms is associated with severe aortic stenosis:

1 Dyspnea: due to decrease cardiac output, decreased LV compliance and elevated LV filling pressures.
2 Chest pain: due to increase demand secondary to hypertrophy, increased afterload and decrease coronary perfusion.
3 Syncope: related to decreased cardiac output and cerebral perfusion.

Etiology

- The most common cause of aortic stenosis is *senile degeneration and calcification* related to age. Mostly seen in patients >75 years of age (Figure 5.1).
- *Bicuspid aortic valve* is the second most common cause of AS after senile degeneration (Figure 5.2). Bicuspid aortic valve is most common cause of AS in patients <75 years of age.
- Rheumatic AS.
- Congenital AS.
- Unicuspid aortic valve.
- Quadricuspid aortic valve (Figure 5.3).

It is important to differentiate valvular aortic stenosis from other causes of LVOT obstruction on echocardiography, as clinical presentation can be similar.

Practical Manual of Echocardiography in the Urgent Setting, First Edition.
Edited by Vladimir Fridman and Mario J. Garcia.
© 2013 John Wiley & Sons, Ltd. Published 2013 by John Wiley & Sons, Ltd.

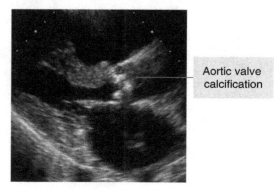

Figure 5.1 Aortic valve with severe calcification.

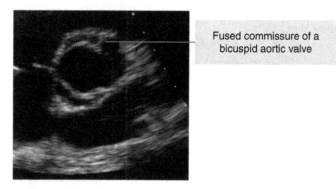

Figure 5.2 Bicuspid aortic valve with a visible fused commissure.

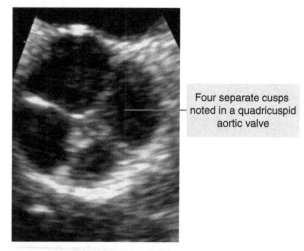

Figure 5.3 Quadricuspid aortic valve.

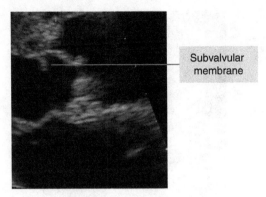

Subvalvular
membrane

Figure 5.4 Subvalvular aortic membrane.

Nonvalvular causes of LVOT obstruction

- Subvalvular (Figure 5.4)

  Subvalvular stenosis is more common than supravalvular.

  a Fixed: Could be due to subvalvular ridge/membrane or tunnel like stenosis. Subvalvular stenosis can cause distortion of aortic valve from high velocity jet coming from subvalvular obstruction that in turn leads to aortic regurgitation.

  b Dynamic: LVOT obstruction in Hypertrophic Cardiomyopathy. Subvalvular obstruction often leads to aortic valve damage due to shear stress by high velocity jet that subsequently leads to aortic regurgitation. The level of obstruction varies at different points in systole.

- Supravalvular

  Supravalvular aortic stenosis is the rarest site of aortic stenosis. Narrowing is seen as either a single discrete constriction or a long tubular narrowing. Associations with Williams syndrome (elfin facies, hypercalcemia and ulmonary stenosis). Sometimes diagnosis may be made by TTE, however most of the time TEE or MRI is required to establish the diagnosis.

Echocardiographic features of aortic stenosis

Echocardiography is the investigation of choice for diagnosis and quantification of aortic stenosis. The following echocardiographic parameters are used for evaluation of aortic stenosis:

- M-mode
- 2D Echocardiography
- Doppler
- M-mode (Figure 5.5)
  - Aortic leaflet separation is calculated during systole (as shown in Chapter 4).
  - Systolic leaflet separation of 15 mm or more by 2D or 2D-guided M-mode echocardiography reliably excludes severe obstruction [1].

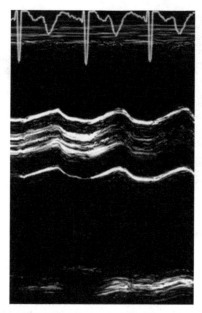

Figure 5.5 M-mode at the level of the aortic valve. The aortic valve is severely calcified, as noted by multiple echodense lines within the valve, and opens poorly in systole.

- ○ Can give clues above etiology of aortic stenosis:
    - ▪ eccentric closure of aortic valve in bicuspid aortic valve;
    - ▪ mid-systolic closure of aortic valve in hypertrophic cardiomyopathy.
  - ○ Figure 5.6 shows normal aortic valve M-mode (a), mild–moderate stenosis (b), and severe stenosis (c).
- • 2D Echocardiography
  - ○ 2D echocardiography is the gold standard in aortic valve evaluation.
  - ○ Allows for differentiation between:
    - ▪ *aortic sclerosis* – thickening and increased echogenicity, especially at the base of the valve leaflets, without significant obstruction.
    - ▪ *aortic stenosis* – calcified aortic valve with reduced opening.
  - ○ Gives clues about etiology of aortic stenosis, such as:
    - ▪ *rheumatic* – diffuse thickening, commissural fusion and mitral valve involvement;
    - ▪ *bicuspid aortic valve* – two cusps instead of three and systolic doming of aortic valve;
    - ▪ unicuspid/quadricuspid aortic valve.
  - ○ Planimetry by 2D echo is also helpful for calculation of aortic valve area. Parasternal short axis view at the base is used for this purpose.

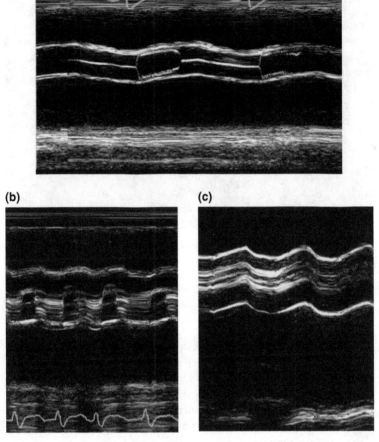

Figure 5.6 M-mode of the aortic valve showing normal valve **(a)**, mild–moderate stenosis **(b)**, and severe stenosis **(c)**.

Sometimes planimetry on TTE imaging may be inaccurate if there is dense calcification of the valve.
  ○ Other than aortic valve structure, 2D echo also gives information about LV size, wall thickness, systolic function, atrial size, mitral valve anatomy and pulmonary artery pressure by Doppler. Surgical treatment is based on some of these measurements.
- Doppler echocardiography
  ○ Used for quantification of aortic stenosis: the higher the velocity through the aortic valve, the higher the pressure gradient, the more severe the stenosis;

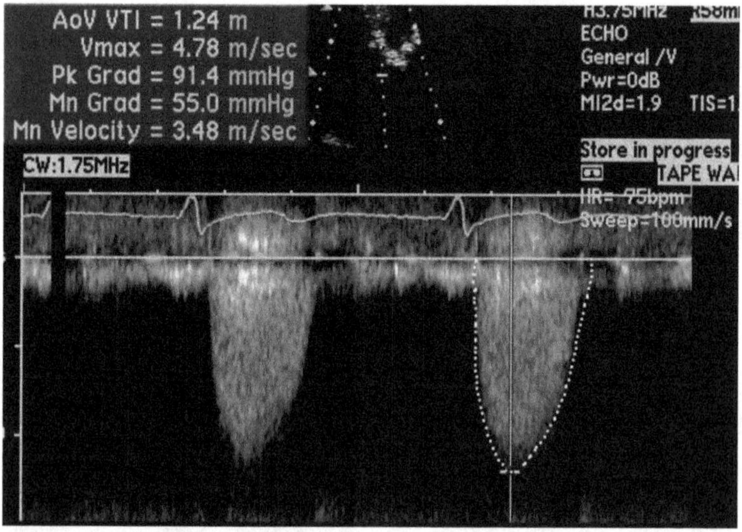

```
AoV VTI = 1.24 m                    H3.75MHz  x58m
    Vmax = 4.78 m/sec               ECHO
  Pk Grad = 91.4 mmHg               General /V
  Mn Grad = 55.0 mmHg               Pwr=0dB
Mn Velocity = 3.48 m/sec            MI2d=1.9  TIS=1
CW:1.75MHz                          Store in progress
                                         TAPE WA
                                    HR= 75bpm
                                    Sweep=100mm/s
```

Figure 5.7 CW Doppler through the aortic valve. When the VTI is traced, the values of the tracing show the presence of severe aortic stenosis.

○ The following measurements are made by Doppler studies:

Peak gradient
▪ Calculated by CW Doppler
▪ Cursor is placed through the opening of the aortic valve in apical three- or five-chamber views (Figure 5.7).
▪ Always use dedicated CW Doppler and multiple windows to obtain maximum velocity if AS is suspected. This is the method to get the true aortic valve velocity–time integral (VTI), through which most of the aortic stenosis calculations are performed.
▪ It is important to use a nonimaging (Pedoff) probe in situations where the optimal angle of incidence cannot be found with an imaging transducer. The correct positioning of this probe is guided by the actual VTI signal that it produces (Figure 5.8).
▪ Peak gradient is measured from peak velocity by using modified Bernoulli equation:

$$\text{Peak gradient} = 4\left(V_{max}\right)^2$$

For example, if peak velocity is 4 m/s, peak gradient will be 64 mmHg.
Note: if LVOT velocity exceeds 1.5 m/s, then $4((V_{max})^2 - (LVOT_{max})^2)$ should be used.

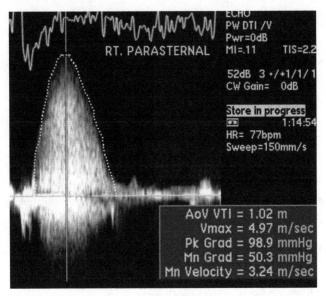

Figure 5.8 Doppler tracing using a nonimaging (Pedoff) probe. Compared to the Figure 5.2 (same patient), the nonimaging probe is usually more accurate, and provides higher gradients, then the CW probe.

Table 5.1 Grading of aortic valve stenosis.

	Aortic stenosis			
	Sclerosis	Mild	Moderate	Severe
Aortic jet velocity (m/s)	≤2.5	2.6–2.9	3.0–4.0	>4
Aortic jet peak gradient (mm Hg)	≤25	26–35	36–64	>64
Mean gradient (mmHg)		<20	20–40	>40
AVA (cm²)		>1.5	1.0–1.5	<1.0
Indexed AVA (cm²/m²)		>0.85	0.6–0.85	<0.6
Velocity ratio (LVOT/AV)		>0.5	0.25–0.5	<0.25

Mean gradient
- Can be calculated by equation:

$$\text{Mean gradient} = 2.4\left(V_{max}\right)^2$$

- V_{max} is maximum peak velocity. Echocardiography machines are programmed to calculate peak and mean gradient automatically from peak velocity (Table 5.1).
- Can also be calculated by tracing the VTI of the flow through the aortic valve (Figure 5.7).

Continuity valve area
- Valve area is calculated by the continuity equation. The continuity equation is based on the law of conservation of mass. In other words, flow across one cardiac chamber is same as across any other in the absence of regurgitation or shunt. That means flow across the LVOT is same as across the aortic valve.
- The continuity equation is derived from the hydraulic formula:

Flow = Area × Flow velocity or $Flow_{LVOT} = CSA_{LVOT} \times VTI_{LVOT}$

Flow across the aortic valve = Flow across the LVOT or

$CSA_{AV} \times VTI_{AV} = CSA_{LVOT} \times VTI_{LVOT}$ or
$CSA_{AV} = CSA_{LVOT} \times VTI_{LVOT} / VTI_{A}$

[CSA (cross-sectional area), LVOT (left ventricular outflow tract), and AV (aortic valve).]

Three measurements are needed to calculate the aortic valve area:

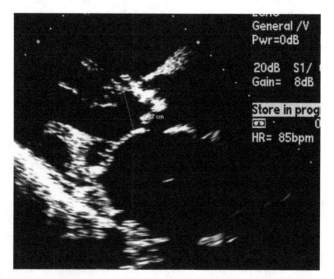

Figure 5.9 Measurement of LVOT diameter in the PLAX view. Note the severe calcifications of the aortic valve leaflets.

i LVOT cross-sectional area is calculated by measuring LVOT diameter at end systole (Figure 5.9). CSA is calculated by following equation:

$$A = \pi r^2 \text{ or } CSA = \pi \left(\frac{D}{2}\right)^2$$

ii LVOT VTI is calculated by using pulse wave Doppler at left ventricular outflow tract in apical window. The cursor is placed just immediately below the aortic valve toward the LVOT, as shown in Figure 5.10.

iii Aortic valve VTI (AV_{VTI}) is calculated by using continuous wave Doppler (Figure 5.7). The cursor is placed at or just above the aortic valve. It is important to measure velocities in different windows to obtain maximum velocity for proper measurements of valve area.

$$\text{Aortic valve area} = \pi \left(\frac{D}{2}\right)^2 \times VTI_{LVOT} / VTI_{AV}$$

Of note:

- Good correlation has been found between the echocardiographic derived valve area and the area calculated by invasive measurements such as cardiac catheterization [2, 3].
- The continuity equation cannot be used in case of hypertrophic cardiomyopathy and subaortic membrane because the effective

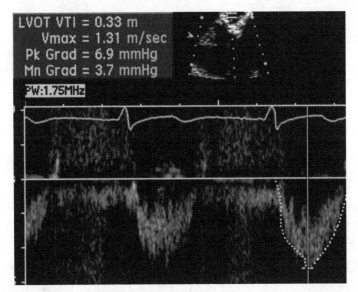

Figure 5.10 Tracing of the LVOT VTI using the PW Doppler.

Table 5.2 AVR surgery indications.

Class/Indication	Level of evidence
Class I	
AVR is indicated for symptomatic patients with severe AS	B
AVR is indicated for patients with severe AS undergoing coronary artery bypass graft surgery.	C
AVR is indicated for patients with severe AS undergoing surgery on the aorta or other heart valves	C
AVR is recommended for patients with severe AS and LV systolic dysfunction (EF <50%)	C
Class IIa	
AVR is reasonable for patients with moderate AS undergoing CABG or surgery on the aorta or other heart valves	B
Class IIb	
AVR may be considered for asymptomatic patients with severe AS and abnormal response to exercise	C
AVR may be considered for adulats with severe asymptomatic AS if there is a high likelihood of rapid progression or if surgery might be delayed at time of symptom onset	C
AVR may be considered in patients undergoing CABG who have mild AS when there is evidence, such as moderate to severe valve calcification, that progression may be rapid	C
AVR may be considered for asymptomatic patients with extremely severe AS (AVA <0.6 cm^2, mean gradient greater than 60 mm Hg, and jet velocity greater than 5 mps) when the patient's expected operative mortality is 1% or less.	C
Class III	
AVR is not useful for the prevention of sudden death in asymptomatic patients with AS who have none of the findings listed under Class IIa/IIb recommendations.	B
Aortic balloon valvotomy	
Class IIb	
Aortic balloon valvotomy might be reasonable as a bridge to surgery in hemodynamically unstable adult patients with AS who are at high risk for AVR.	C

Table 5.2 (Cont'd)	
Class/Indication	**Level of evidence**
Aortic balloon valvotomy might be reasonable for palliation in adult patients with AS in whom AVR cannot be performed because of serious comorbid conditions	C
Class III	
Aortic balloon valvotomy is not recommended as an alternative to AVR in adulat patients with AS; certain younger adults without valve calcification may be an exception.	B

LVOT is not circular or the velocity exceeds Nyquist limit in these conditions.

Velocity ratio (dimensionless index)
- The velocity ratio ($LVOT_{VTI}:AV_{VTI}$) of the left ventricular out flow tract and aortic valve can give an estimation of the severity of aortic stenosis.
- A velocity ratio <0.25 indicates severe aortic stenosis.

All of the values for mild, moderate, and severe aortic stenosis are shown in Table 5.1.

- It is often difficult to determine the severity of aortic stenosis in patients with reduced LV stroke volume. These patients appear to have moderate stenosis on the basis of mean gradients, while severe aortic stenosis on the basis of continuity valve area. By increasing LV contractility and stroke volume using intravenous dobutamine it is often possible to differentiate moderate from severe AS:
  i The aortic valve area by continuity and the mean gradient are measured at rest.
  ii These measurements are repeated with dobutamine infusion, starting with low dose of 5µg/kg/min up to a maximum dose of 20µg/kg/min.
  iii Constant valve area with increase in gradients suggests severe aortic stenosis.
  iv Increase in valve area with insignificant increase in gradients suggests primary myocardial dysfunction.

Treatment of aortic stenosis is outside of the scope of this book. However, the indications for surgical intervention in cases of aortic stenosis are shown in Table 5.2 [4].

Aortic regurgitation

Aortic regurgitation (AR) may have an acute or a chronic presentation and may be caused by a variety of conditions. AR severity is determined by the volume of aortic regurgitation, and by the hemodynamic effects of the volume overload on the left ventricle. It is important to determine both the cause and severity of aortic regurgitation to guide the treatment of these patients.

The hemodynamic effects of aortic regurgitation are largely based on the acuity of regurgitation. Acute vesus chronic aortic insufficiency (AI) are very different clinical syndromes, and have very different presentations and treatments. In acute severe AI, the regurgitant jet might have a short duration due to the rapid rise of LV pressure in diastole. Chronic regurgitation is associated more with a dilated left ventricle and with lower interventricular pressures than those of acute regurgitation. Clinically, acute severe aortic regurgitation patients present with severe heart failure and possibly cardiogenic shock. Chronic AI patients can present with heart failure symptoms, but in most cases these are gradual in onset and respond to medical treatment.

Whether acute or chronic, treatment still depends on the severity of the regurgitation. There are many echocardiographic parameters that help establish severity of aortic regurgitation (Figure 5.11).

(a)

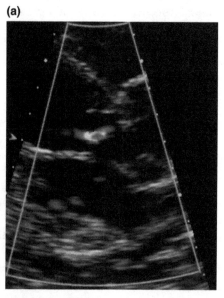

Figure 5.11 Qualitative measurement of aortic insufficiency: **(a)** mild AI in PLAX view; **(b)** moderate AI in PLAX view; **(c)** severe AI in the apical three-chamber view.

(b)

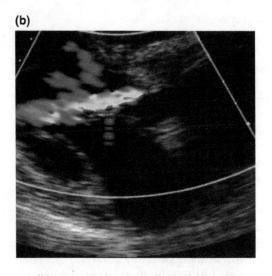

(c)

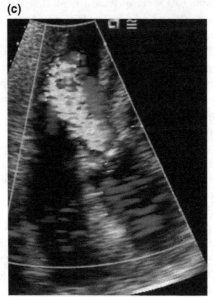

Figure 5.11 (*Cont'd*)

Common causes of aortic regurgitation are:
- Congenital malformation of aortic valve (bicuspid, unicuspid, quadricuspid)
- Rheumatic heart disease
- Syphilitic aortitis
- Ankylosing spondylitis

- Rheumatoid arthiritis
- Marfan's syndrome, and other abnormalities of connective tissues
- Infective endocarditis
- Annuloaortic ectasia
- Trauma
- Aortic dissection
- Malfunction of aortic valve prosthesis.

In acute aortic insufficiency, the common diagnoses that must be ruled out are:

- Endocarditis
- Aortic dissection
- Prosthetic valve malfunction (if clinical scenario is correct) [5].

Prior to starting the process of determining the severity of AI, it is extremely important to get accurate measurements of the LV thickness and dimensions, in systole and diastole. These are important later on when the course of treatment for aortic regurgitation needs to selected.

When determining AI severity, there are multiple specific echocardiographic measurements and calculations that must be performed.

- Vena contracta width

  In parasternal long axis view, color Doppler is applied to the aortic valve area including a few centimeters into the LV cavity. Then the picture is paused and the diameter of the AI jet is taken at its narrowest point just distal to the aortic valve in the LVOT (the vena contracta) (Figure 5.12).

- Regurgitation jet width/LVOT diameter ratio

  In parasternal long axis view, color Doppler is applied to the aortic valve area including a few centimeters into the LV cavity. An M-mode image is taken at the point in the LVOT where the AI jet is the widest. Then, in M-mode imaging, the diameter of the LVOT and the diameter of the AI jet are taken, and their diameter ratio is determined.

- Aortic regurgitation pressure half time

  In either the apical five-chamber or three-chamber views, color Doppler is applied to the aortic valve area including a few centimeters into the LV cavity. Then a CW Doppler image is taken through the AI jet. A good AI jet picture shows a smooth deceleration curve of the jet (Figures 5.13

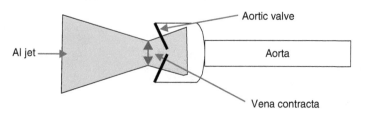

Figure 5.12 Measurement of the vena contracta.

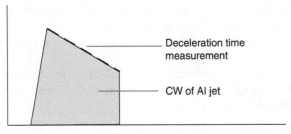

Figure 5.13 Representation of a CW Doppler image of aortic regurgitation jet.

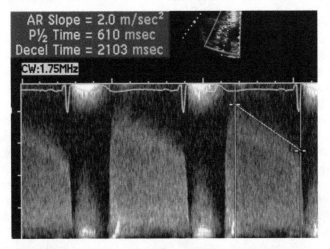

Figure 5.14 CW Doppler image of aortic regurgitation jet.

and 5.14). Using the calculations menu in the echocardiography machine, a line is drawn from the peak of the AI jet in the beginning to the trough of the AI jet at the end. This slope is then used to calculate the deceleration time of the AI jet, which then is converted to the pressure ½ measurement by:

$P\frac{1}{2} = 0.29 \times$ deceleration time

- Aortic regurgitation volume
  - The volumetric method for AI assumes that the volume of forward flow that goes through the LVOT (and thus through the aortic valve) minus the volume of forward flow that goes through the mitral valve (MV) is equal to the aortic regurgitation volume.

MV inflow = Mitral valve annulus area × Mitral valve VTI

LVOT inflow = LVOT area × LVOT VTI

○ The Proximal Isovelocity Surface Area (PISA) method can also be used to calculate the volume of the AI jet.
  • The same PISA formula is applied in AI as in mitral regurgitation (MR) (discussed later in this chapter).
  • The effective regurgitant orifice (ERO) is calculated-where the only change in formula is that the peak AI jet velocity instead of MR velocity is used.

Regurgitant volume = ERO × AI$_{VTI}$

○ Regurgitation Fraction of the AI jet

RF = Aortic regurgitation volume / LVOT forward flow volume × 100

• Reversal of flow in the descending aorta
This can be assessed by color or pulsed Doppler, from the suprasternal notch or the subcostal view. Severe AR is characterized by holodiastolic flow reversal with a maximal velocity of 0.5 m/s and a terminal velocity of 0.2 m/s or greater.

It is important to take into account all echocardiographic calculations to assess the severity of aortic regurgitation. All the methods listed above have their limitations: the vena contracta jet width and area may underestimate AR severity if the jet is eccentric (bicuspid valves, trauma); the pressure half-time method may overestimate AR severity if there is reduced LV compliance (severe AS); the reversal of flow method may underestimate severity in severe acute AR. The values for mild, moderate, and severe aortic regurgitation are shown in Table 5.3. After the severity of AI is determined, it should then be combined with the clinical presentation of the patient in order to select and begin the proper treatment for the patient [4].

Mitral valve

The mitral valve is a complex structure. It is made of up of the anterior and posterior leaflets, and each of these leaflets has three scallops (labeled 1–3) (Figure 5.15). The anterior leaflet is shorter but wider than the posterior scallop.

The entire mitral valve apparatus is made up of multiple anatomical structures. These are:
• Mitral valve leaflets.
• Mitral valve annulus.
• Chordae tendinae, connecting the mitral valve leaflets to the papillary muscles.
• Papillary muscles.
• Portions of the left atrium and left ventricle where the mitral valve attaches.

Table 5.3 Grading of aortic valve insufficiency.

	Aortic Regurgitation		
	Mild	Moderate	Severe
Structural parameters			
LA size	normal	normal or dilated	usually dilated
Aortic leaflets	normal or abnormal	normal or abnormal	abnormal/ flail, or wide coaptation defect
Doppler Parameters			
Jet width in LVOT-Color Flow	Small in central jets	Intermediate	Large in central jets; variable in eccentric jets
Jet Density-CW	Incomplete or faint	Dense	Dense
Jet deceleration rate-CW (PHT, ms)	Slow >500	Medium 500–200	Steep <200
Diastolic flow reversal in descending aorta-PW	Brief, early diastolic reversal	Intermediate	Prominent holodiastolic reversal
Quantitative parameters			
VC width (cm)	<0.3	0.3–0.6	>0.6
Jet width/LVOT width (%)	<25	25–45; 46–64	≥65
Jet CSA/LVOT CSA (%)	<5	5–20; 21–59	≥60
R Vol (ml/beat)	<30	30–44; 45–59	≥60
RF (%)	<30	30–39; 40–49	≥50
EROA (cm^2)	<0.10	0.10–0.19; 0.20–0.29	≥0.30

Mitral valve incompetence can arise from pathologies involving any of the above named parts. On echocardiography, all of these segments of the mitral valve apparatus need to be evaluated in order to conclude whether the mitral valve is or is not involved in the clinical syndrome of the patient.

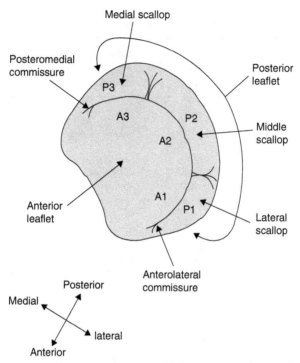

Figure 5.15 Anatomy of the mitral valve (Reproduced from Shanewise *et al.* [6], with permission from Elsevier).

Mitral stenosis

Mitral stenosis (MS) is a condition characterized by the narrowing of the opening of the mitral valve. The most common cause of mitral stenosis is rheumatic heart disease. However, other causes include severe annular calcification and congenital abnormalities. On 2D echocardiography, mitral stenosis has multiple important findings.

- In rheumatic disease, on parasternal long axis view, the valve opens only slightly and the anterior leaflet of the mitral valve appears to resemble a "hockey stick" (Figure 5.16).
- In rheumatic disease, on parasternal short axis view at the mitral valve level, the maximum mitral valve opening is small (fish mouth appearance) and planimetry at this level indicates a small mitral valve area.
- Usually, the left ventricle is small and the left atrium is dilated.
- When the mitral valve stenosis is from severe calcification, the valve on echocardiography appears severely calcified with very

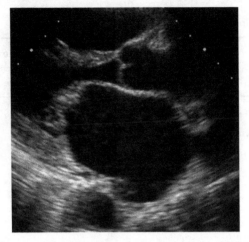

Figure 5.16 Parasternal long axis view of mitral valve stenosis. Note the thickening of the mitral valve leaflets, and the anterior leaflet resembles a "hockey stick".

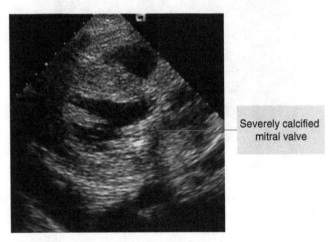

Severely calcified
mitral valve

Figure 5.17 Severely calcified mitral valve.

small excursion of the valve leaflets throughout the cardiac cycle (Figure 5.17).

There are multiple quantitative ways to determine severity of the mitral stenosis. Table 5.4 shows the values for mild, moderate, and severe mitral stenosis.

Table 5.4 Grading of mitral valve stenosis.

	Mitral Stenosis		
	Mild	Moderate	Severe
Specific findings			
Valve area (cm²)	>1.5	1.0–1.5	<1.0
Supportive findings			
Mean gradient (mm Hg)	<5	5–10	>10
Pulmonary artery pressure (mm Hg)	<30	30–50	>50

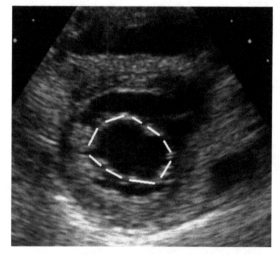

Figure 5.18 Planimetry of the mitral valve in parasternal short axis view at the mitral valve level.

- Planimetry – in the parasternal short axis view at the mitral valve level, planimetry of the entire mitral valve opening will give the mitral valve area (Figure 5.18). This is the most reliable method if there is good image quality and the valve calcification is limited.
- Pressure half-time (PHT) method
  - A CW Doppler is taken through the mitral valve opening.
  - A characteristic mitral inflow is obtained when MS is present (Figure 5.19).

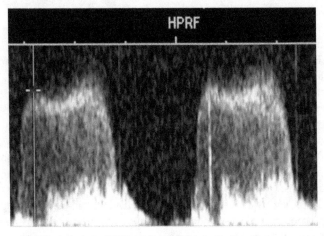

Figure 5.19 Characteristic CW Doppler profile of mitral stenosis.

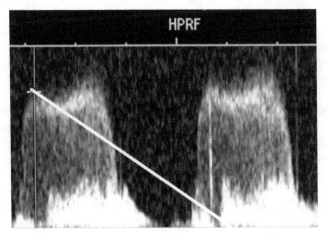

Figure 5.20 Drawing of deceleration line on mitral stenosis Doppler profile.

- A line is drawn from the highest initial deflection (E point) to the baseline with the slope being the decreasing velocity Doppler signal (Figure 5.20).
- The echocardiogram machine calculation package will compute the pressure ½ time for this deceleration lime (Pressure half time = 0.29 × deceleration time).
- Mitral valve area = 220 / pressure half time.

- Gradient
  - The CW Doppler tracing used for PHT method is used in this method.
  - Tracing this CW Doppler signal will give the mitral valve inflow VTI and the mean mitral valve gradient.
- Continuity valve area

  In the absence if significant valvular regurgitation, the mitral valve area can be calculated as: $MVA = SV_{LVOT} / MV_{VTI}$.
- Pulmonary artery systolic pressure
  - As will be seen in the MS management algorithm, diagnosing pulmonary hypertension is extremely important in cases of mitral stenosis.
  - Based on the guidelines (as presented later in this chapter), pulmonary artery systolic pressures are important to measure during exercise as well as in certain mitral stenosis cases. This can be achieved with stress echocardiography.

It is important to take into account that there are many clinical scenarios in which the results of these methods may be discrepant:

- The gradients may be reduced in patients with bradycardia and low cardiac output and conversely increased in the opposite conditions.
- The pressure half time is influenced by the compliance of the LV and the LA; therefore, mitral stenosis severity may be underestimated if there is concomitant severe aortic stenosis or severely increased LA pressure.
- The calculation of MV area by continuity may underestimate the severity of mitral stenosis in the presence of significant AR or overestimate it in the presence of significant MR.

Besides lowering heart rate and the use of diuretics to control symptoms, mitral stenosis is treated by valvotomy or valve replacement.

Whether a specific mitral valve is amenable to balloon valvotomy is determined by the Wilkins score [7]. The Wilkins score system is shown in Table 5.5 and involves the grading of four mitral valve anatomy factors on a scale of 1–4. These anatomy factors are:

- Mitral valve leaflet mobility
- Mitral valve leaflet thickening
- Mitral valve calcification
- Subvalvular thickening.

Patients with scores of >8 have been shown to have high rates of acute mitral insufficiency and/or persistent mitral valve stenosis post valvotomy, and the percutaneous procedure is not recommended. It is also important to note that the presence of concomitant moderate or severe mitral regurgitation (any mitral regurgitation above 2+) is a contraindication to mitral valve balloon valvotomy.

Table 5.5 Wilkins score for mitral valve stenosis [7].

Grade	Mobility	Thickening	Calcification	Subvalvular thickening
1	Highly mobile valve with only leaflet tips restricted	Leaflets near normal in thickness (4–5 mm)	A single area of increased echo brightness	Minimal thickening just below the mitral leaflets
2	Leaflet mid and base portions have normal mobility	Midleaflets normal, considerable thickening of margins (5–8 mm)	Scattered areas of brightness confined to leaflet margins	Thickening of chordal structures extending to one-third of the chordal length
3	Valve continues to move forward in diastole, mainly from the base	Thickening extending through the entire leaflet (5–8 mm)	Brightness extending into the mid-portions of the leaflets	Thickening extended to distal third of the chords
4	No or minimal forward movements of the leaflets in diastole	Considerable thickening of all leaflet tissue (>8–10 mm)	Extensive brightness throughout much of the leaflet tissue	Extensive thickening and shortening of all chordal structures extending down to the papillary muscles

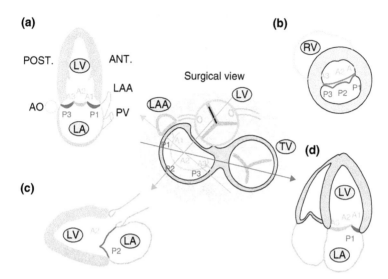

Figure 5.21 Mitral valve scallops visualized in different TTE views: **(a)** apical two-chamber views; **(b)** parasternal short axis view; **(c)** parasternal long axis view; **(d)** apical four-chamber view (Reproduced from Monin *et al.* [8], with permission from Elsevier).

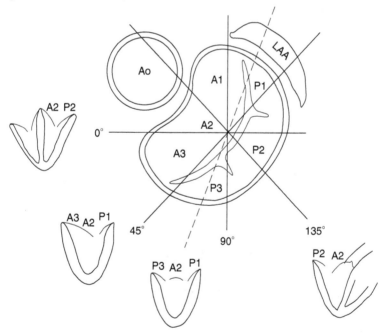

Figure 5.22 TEE views of mitral valve scallops (Reproduced from Foster *et al.* [9], with permission from Elsevier).

Mitral regurgitation

Mitral regurgitation (MR) is a common clinical disorder that can have many causes and many treatment pathways. Visualization of the entire mitral valve apparatus is also extremely difficult in echocardiography, and often requires TEE. However, any echocardiographer should be able to identify the mechanism and severity of mitral regurgitation by TTE in most clinical scenarios.

As discussed earlier, the mitral valve has two leaflets, which are split into six scallops. On different TTE views, various scallops can be visualized:

- Figure 5.21 shows the different scallops that are seen on a transthoracic echocardiogram [8].
- Figure 5.22 shows which scallops of the mitral valve are visualized in different TEE views [9].
- Figure 5.23 shows the different views of the mitral valve that are obtained by moving the TEE probe in various directions [9].

Mitral regurgitation can be an acute or a chronic (compensated or decompensated) process. Acute mitral regurgitation usually involves hemodynamic compromise (if severe) as the ventricle and atria have not had the time to adjust to the increased volume load. Chronic mitral regurgitation is a hemodynamically stable process as the left sided chambers have adjusted to the effects of mitral regurgitation over time.

Causes of mitral regurgitation are:

- Ischemic mitral regurgitation, which may be chronic or acute, including papillary muscle rupture.
- Rupture of chordae tendinae (Figure 5.24).
- Mitral valve prolapse – when the mitral valve leaflet is displaced >2 mm in systole above the mitral annulus plane (Figure 5.25).
- Endocarditis.
- Rheumatic fever.
- Dilated cardiomyopathy.
- Drug induced

The direction of mitral regurgitation can aid in diagnosing of the cause of the regurgitation:

- Jet of mitral valve prolapse flows away from the prolapsed leaflet.
- Jet of mitral regurgitation due to tethering of a mitral valve leaflet produces regurgitation toward the side of the tethered leaflet. If both leaflets are tethered, a central jet is produced.
- Ischemic mitral regurgitation is caused by tethering of the leaflet which is connected to an ischemic area, and is thus directed toward this leaflet.

Once the presence of mitral regurgitation is noted, its severity has to be determined (Figure 5.26). There are multiple ways to determine the severity of mitral valve regurgitation.

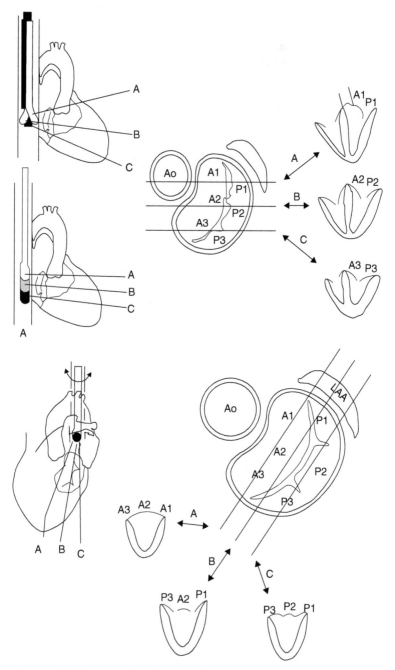

Figure 5.23 TEE views of mitral valve scallops as the probe is moved in various directions: **(a)** effect of flexion or retroflexion and advancement or withdrawal of the probe; **(b)** effect of clockwise and counterclockwise rotation of the probe (Reproduced from Foster *et al.* [9], with permission from Elsevier).

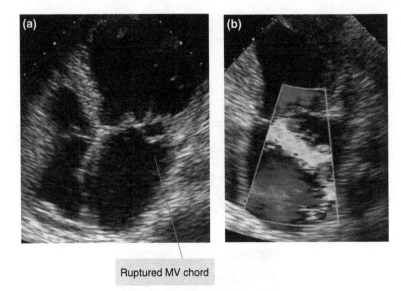

Figure 5.24 (a) Presence of a ruptured mitral valve chord in the apical four-chamber view, and **(b)** resultant severe mitral regurgitation.

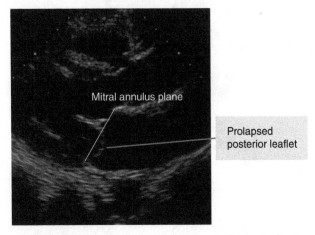

Figure 5.25 Prolapse of the posterior leaflet of the mitral valve is clearly noted in this PLAX view.

- Volumetric
  - Volume of MR = Volume going from the LA to the LV in diastole (mitral valve inflow) – volume of flow going through the LVOT in systole (LVOT inflow)

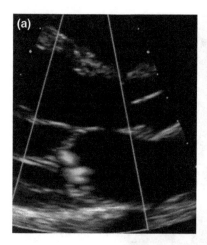
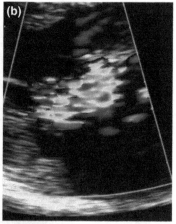
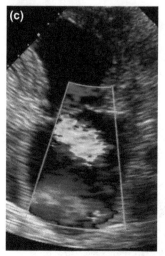

Figure 5.26 Qualitative assessment of mitral regurgitation: **(a)** mild MR in PLAX view; **(b)** moderate MR in PLAX view; **(c)** severe MR in apical two-chamber view.

- ○ Volume of MV inflow = MV area × MV VTI
- ○ Volume of LVOT inflow = LVOT area × LVOT VTI
- Regurgitant fraction
  - ○ MR Regurgitant fraction = MR volume / Mitral valve inflow × 100
- Vena contracta width
  - ○ Similar to calculating vena contracta width in AR.
  - ○ Color Doppler is used to view the MR jet in parasternal long axis view.
  - ○ The diameter of the regurgitation jet at its narrowest point, a few millimeters distal to the mitral valve leaflets into the LA, is the vena contracta width.

- Area of the mitral regurgitation jet
  - ○ The percentage of left atrial area that is taken up by the MR jet is a measure of severity.
  - ○ Planimetry of the MR jet using color Doppler as guide is a measure of severity.
  - ○ These measures are not extremely accurate as it depends on the Doppler gain setting, and also can underestimate the jet if it hugs the wall of the left atrium (Coanda effect).
- Proximal Isovelocity Surface Area (PISA) method
  - ○ The step-by-step guide to this calculation is shown in Box 5.1.
  - ○ The appearance of an appropriate PISA hemispheric shell is seen in Figure 5.27, with its radius labeled "r" [10].

Box 5.1 Step-by-step guide to performing a PISA calculation for mitral regurgitation.

$$MR\ Volume = MR\ ROA \times MR\ VTI$$

Step 1: In apical four-chamber view, zoom in on the mitral valve.

Step 2: Place color Doppler on the mitral valve so that a good portion of the ventricle and left atrium next to the mitral valve is imaged by the Doppler.

Step 3: Attempt to identify the PISA hemispheric shell – this is the most difficult part of the calculation. This will be on the LV side of the mitral valve, as flow is going from the LV to the LA.

- To make the PISA shell clearer, shift the baseline or scale so that the flow going away from the probe aliases at a lower velocity. Sometimes this is referred to as "shifting baseline toward the flow".
- Attempt to make slight changes in the baseline or scale of the Doppler until a clear hemispheric shell is visualized that is uniform in color on the inside and changes color (aliases) on its outer border.

Step 4: Once a PISA shell is clearly seen, pause the echo image and record the PISA shell radius.

Step 5: In apical view, record the CW Doppler of the MR jet. Record the MR jet VTI in systole.

Step 6: To measure regurgitant fraction, flow through mitral valve in diastole should also be recorded. Zoom in on the mitral valve. Record the mitral valve diameter.

Step 7: Record the PW Doppler of the mitral valve – the cursor should be placed at the level of the mitral valve annulus. Record the VTI of the mitral valve in diastole (if aliasing is present, record CW instead of PW).

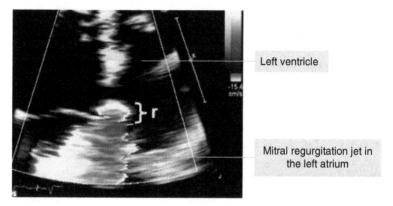

Figure 5.27 PISA hemispheric shell with its radius labeled "r" (Reproduced from Buck *et al.* [10], with permission from Elsevier).

○ The important part of this calculation is to differentiate between the various formulas and values involved. It is necessary to keep in mind which formulas need peak velocity and which formulas need TVI.

- Flow rate = Area × Velocity
- Volume = Area × TVI
- ERO (effective regurgitant orifice) = $(2\pi r^2 \times$ PISA Aliasing V$)$ / MR peak velocity
- MR volume = ERO × MR VTI
- As a shortcut, if the PISA aliasing velocity is set to 40 cm/s, and the peak velocity of the MR jet is approximately 5 m/s (can be assumed under if the patient has normal blood pressure and does not have clinical signs of elevated left atrial pressures), the ERO formula is simplified to:

$$ERO = r^2 / 2$$

All of these measurements should be used together to determine the severity of mitral regurgitation. The cutoffs for mild, moderate, and severe mitral regurgitation are shown in Table 5.6.

For a comprehensive review of the indications and guidelines for management of valvular heart disease, the ACC/AHA guidelines, initially published in 2006 and updated in 2008, should be referred to [4].

The treatment of mitral regurgitation depends on the acuity, severity, and hemodynamic significance of the regurgitation. Guidelines for mitral valve surgery are shown in Table 5.7, and the management strategy for chronic severe mitral regurgitation is available in the ACC/AHA guidelines [4].

Table 5.6 Grading of mitral valve regurgitation.

	Mitral regurgitation		
	Mild	Moderate	Severe
Specific signs of severity	Small central jet <4 cm² or <20% of LA area	Signs of MR > mild present, but no criteria for severe MR	Vena contracta width ≥0.7 cm with large central MR jet (area >40% of LA) or with a wall-impinging jet of any size, swirling in LA
	Vena contracta width <0.3 cm	–	Large flow convergence
	No or minimal flow convergence	–	Systolic reversal in pulmonary veins
	–	–	Prominent flail MV leaflet or ruptured papillary muscle
Supportive signs of severity	Systolic dominant flow in pulmonary veins	Intermediate signs/findings	Dense, triangular CW Doppler MR jet
	A-wave dominant mitral inflow	–	E-wave dominant mitral inflow (E>1.2 m/s). Enlarged LV and LA, (particularly when normal LV function is present)
	Soft density, parabolic CW Doppler MR signal		
	Normal LV size		
R Vol (ml/beat)	<30	30–44; 45–59	≥60
RF (%)	<30	30–39; 40–49	≥50
EROA (cm²)	<0.2	0.2–0.29; 0.3–0.39	≥0.4

Table 5.7 Mitral regurgitation surgery indications.

Class/Indication	Level of evidence
Class I	
MV surgery is recommended for the symptomatic patient with acute severe MR	B
MV surgery is beneficial for patients with chronic severe MR and NYHA functional class II, III, or IV symptoms in the absence of severe LV dysfunction (EF <30%) and/or end-systolic dimension >55 mm.	B
MV surgery is beneficial for asymptomatic patients with chronic severe MR and mild to moderate LV dysfunction, EF between 30% and 60%, and/or end-systolic dimension greater ≥40 mm.	B
MV repair is recommended over MV replacement in the majority of patients with severe chronic MR who require surgery, and patients should be referred to surgical center experienced in MV repair.	C
Class IIa	
MV repair is reasonable in experienced surgical centers for asymptomatic patients with chronic severe MR with preserved LV function (LV >60% and end-systolic dimension <40 mm) in whom the likelihood of successful repair without residual MR is >90%.	B
MV surgery is reasonable for asymptomatic patients with chronic severe MR, preserved LV function, and new onset of atrial fibrillation.	C
MV surgery is reasonable for asymptomatic patients with chronic severe MR, preserved LV function, and pulmonary hypertension (pulmonary artery systolic pressure greater than 50 mmHg at rest or greater than 60 mm Hg with exercise).	C
MV surgery is reasonable for patients with chronic severe MR due to a primary abnormality of the mitral apparatus and NYHA functional class III-IV symptoms and severe LV dysfunction (EF <30% and/or end-systolic dimension >55 mm) in whom MV repair is highly likely.	C
Class IIb	
MV repair may be considered for patients with chronic severe secondary MR due to severe LV dysfunction (EF <30%) who have persistent NYHA functional class III-IV symptoms despite optimal therapy for heart failure, including biventricular pacing.	C

Table 5.7 (*Cont'd*)

Class/Indication	Level of evidence
Class III	
MV surgery is not indicated for asymptomatic patients with MR and preserved LV function (EF>60% and end-systolic dimension <40 mm) in whom significant doubt about the feasibility of repair exists.	C
Isolated MV surgery is not indicated for patients with mild or moderate MR.	C

In summary, a full evaluation of left sided cardiac valves is necessary with every echocardiogram. All stenotic or regurgitation lesions must be evaluated qualitatively and quantitatively. However, echocardiographic evaluation of right sided valves is also extremely important; this is discussed in the next chapter.

References

1 Otto, C. *Textbook of Clinical Echocardiography*. Philadelphia: WB Saunders Co, 2009.
2 Skjaerpe T, Hegrenaes L, Hatle L. Noninvasive estimation of valve area in patients with aortic stenosis by Doppler ultrasound and two-dimensional echocardiography. *Circulation* 1985; 72:810–8.
3 Oh JK, Taliercio CP, Holmes DR Jr, *et al*. Prediction of the severity of aortic stenosis by Doppler aortic valve area determination: Prospective Doppler-catheterization correlation in 100 patients. *J Am Coll Cardiol* 1988; 11:1227–34.
4 Bonow RO, Carabello BA, Chatterjee K, *et al*. 2008 Focused update incorporated into the ACC/AHA 2006 guidelines for the management of patients with valvular heart disease. *J Am Coll Cardiol* 2008; 52(13):1–142.
5 Jamet B, Chabert JP, Metz D, Elaerts J. Acute Aortic Insufficiency. *Ann Cardiol Angeiol* 2000; 49(3):183–6.
6 Shanewise JS, Cheung AT, Aronson S, *et al*. ASE/SCA guidelines for performing a comprehensive intraoperative multiplane transesophageal echocardiography examination: Recommendations of the American Society of Echocardiography Council for Intraoperative Echocardiography and the Society of Cardiovascular Anesthesiologists Task Force for Certification in Perioperative Transesophageal Echocardiography. *J Am Soc Echocardiogr* 1999; 12:884–900.
7 Palacios IF, Block PC, Wilkins GT, Weyman AE. Follow-up of patients undergoing percutaneous mitral balloon valvotomy. Analysis of factors determining restenosis. *Circulation* 1989; 79:573–9.
8 Monin JL, Dehant P, Roiron C, *et al*. Functional assessment of mitral regurgitation by transthoracic echocardiography using standardized imaging planes: diagnostic accuracy and outcome implications. *J Am Coll Cardiol* 2005; 46(2):302–9.

9 Foster GP, Isselbacher EM, Rose GA, *et al.* Accurate localization of mitral regurgitant defects using multiplane transesophageal echocardiography. *Ann Thorac Surg* 1998; 65(4):1025–31.

10 Buck T, Plicht B, Kahlert P, *et al.* Effect of dynamic flow rate and orifice area on mitral regurgitant stroke volume quantification using the proximal isovelocity surface area method. *J Am Coll Cardiol* 2008; 52(9):767–78.

Right-sided heart valves

Michael J. Levine[1] and Vladimir Fridman[2]

[1]Cardiovascular Diseases, NYU Langone Medical Center,
New York, NY, USA
[2]Cardiovascular Diseases, New York, NY, USA

CHAPTER 6

Even though the right-sided heart valves do not get as much attention as their left counterparts, their careful echocardiographic interrogation remains important. They provide important data on the hemodynamic state of the patient, as well as giving a clear understanding of the function of the right side of the heart. As such, to an echocardiographer knowledge of imaging the right-sided heart valves is absolutely essential.

Tricuspid valve

The tricuspid valve is a complex structure. It consists of the septal, anterior, and posterior leaflets and separates the right atrium from the right ventricle. Due to the complexity of its anatomy, no single two-dimensional transthoracic echocardiographic view can show all of the three leaflets.

However, when multiple views are taken of the tricuspid valve, its anatomic structure and function can be investigated successfully using an echocardiogram. Furthermore, the regurgitation jet of the tricuspid valve is extremely important in hemodynamic measurements, especially of the pulmonary artery systolic pressure.

Views of the tricuspid valve (more detailed explanation in Chapter 2):

- RV inflow view (Figure 6.1): in this view, the anterior and posterior leaflets of the tricuspid valve are visualized. Furthermore, this is a great view to check for any tricuspid regurgitation [1].
- Parasternal short axis view of the base (Figure 6.2): the septal and anterior leaflets are visualized. Also, this is a great view to check for tricuspid regurgitation.

Practical Manual of Echocardiography in the Urgent Setting, First Edition.
Edited by Vladimir Fridman and Mario J. Garcia.

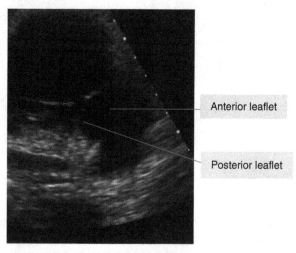

Figure 6.1 RV inflow view and the visible tricuspid valve leaflets.

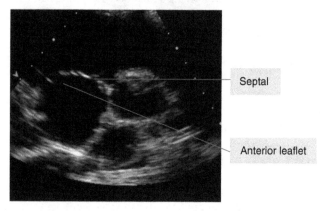

Figure 6.2 Parasternal short axis view of the base and the visible tricuspid valve leaflets.

- Apical four-chamber view (Figure 6.3): the septal and anterior leaflets are visualized. In this view, it is extremely important to check for the location of the tricuspid valve in relation to the mitral valve. The tricuspid valve (mainly the septal leaflet) should be located more apical than the mitral valve, but by no more than 7 mm. Further apical displacement of the tricuspid valve should lead the echocardiographer to consider Ebstein's anomaly.
- The subcostal long axis view can display the anterior and septal leaflets of the tricuspid valve (Figure 6.4a). The subcostal short axis view can show the tricuspid and pulmonic valves (Figure 6.4b).

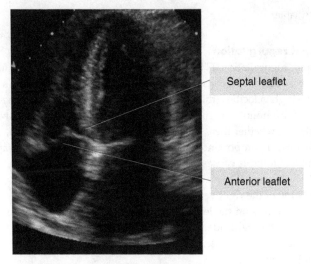

Figure 6.3 Apical four-chamber view and the visible tricuspid valve leaflets.

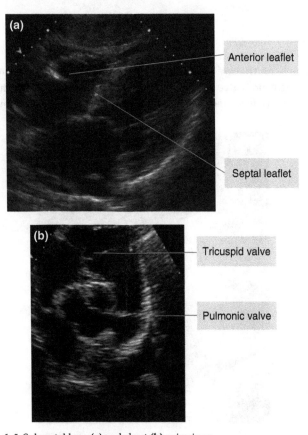

Figure 6.4 Subcostal long **(a)** and short **(b)** axis views.

Tricuspid regurgitation

Tricuspid regurgitation (TR) can be found in more than 50% of the population. For it to be considered "normal", it should be mild and should not have high velocities (thus high pulmonary pressures). Anything more than a small amount of regurgitation is considered pathological. However, regardless of whether there is very minimal or severe regurgitation, the jet velocity provides important hemodynamic data to the echocardiographer.

There are multiple causes of pathological tricuspid regurgitation. These include:
- Dilatation of the right ventricle.
- Any pathology on the left side of the heart that impacts the hemodynamics on the right side.
- Rheumatic heart disease.
- Ebstein's anomaly.
- Carcinoid heart disease.
- Marfan's syndrome.
- Thraumatic injury.
- Radiation therapy.
- Drug induced.

To evaluate for tricuspid regurgitation, color Doppler should be applied to the tricuspid valve and the right atrium in every view that the tricuspid valve is visualized. When the jet is noted (Figures 6.5 and 6.6),

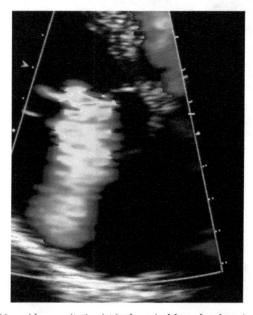

Figure 6.5 Tricuspid regurgitation jet in the apical four-chamber view.

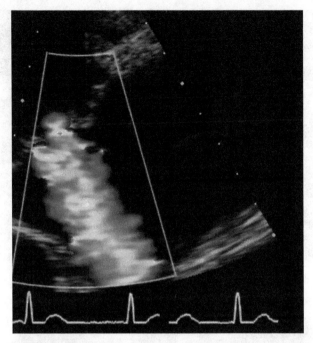

Figure 6.6 Tricuspid regurgitation jet in the RV inflow view.

the CW Doppler should be applied through the highest intensity portion of the jet to get the peak velocity of tricuspid regurgitation (Figure 6.7).

As with prior calculations:

$$4 \times (\text{velocity of TR jet})^2 = \text{gradient between RA and RV}$$

Based on the estimation of the right atrial pressure via IVC measurement (as discussed in Chapter 4), adding RA pressure to the above gradient will give the pulmonary artery systolic pressure.

It is important to keep in mind that in cases of very mild TR, the Doppler signal may be weak. Determination of the right ventricular systolic pressure (RVSP) is unreliable if the full envelope is not defined (Figure 6.8). At the same time, in cases of severe tricuspid regurgitation, the right atrial pressure becomes "ventricularized"; therefore; its estimation is difficult and RVSP tends to be underestimated.

The severity of the tricuspid regurgitant jet also has important clinical significance. As with mitral regurgitation, there are multiple different methods to calculate tricuspid regurgitation severity:

- PISA radius – the same method of determining a Proximal Isovelocity Surface Area (PISA) radius as for the MR jet is used in the calculation of the TR jet severity.

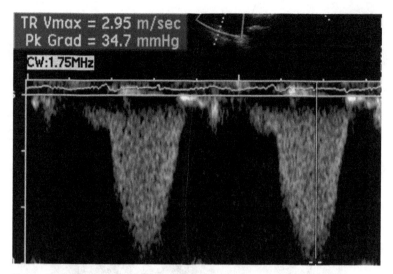

Figure 6.7 CW Doppler of tricuspid regurgitation jet.

(a) **(b)**

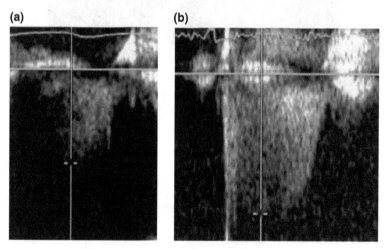

Figure 6.8 CW Doppler TR jet in the same patient. Realignment of the Doppler interrogation line resulted in more complete TR jet envelope and in a clinically significant increase of TR jet V_{max} from 1.3 **(a)** to 2.8 **(b)**.

- Vena contracta – same measurement technique applies as for earlier valves.
- CW intensity – when compared to the intensity of the tricuspid valve inflow signal, if the regurgitation jet is:
  - ○ Much less intense – mild TR
  - ○ Slightly less intense – moderate TR
  - ○ Same intensity – severe TR

Table 6.1 Tricuspid regurgitation.

	Tricuspid regurgitation		
	Mild	**Moderate**	**Severe**
Tricuspid valve	Usually normal	Normal or abnormal	Abnormal/flail leaflet/poor coaptation
RV/RA/IVC size	Normal	Normal or dilated	Usually dilated
Jet area-central jets (cm²)	<5	5–10	>10
VC width (cm)	Not defined	Not defined, but <0.7	>0.7
PISA radium (cm)	≤0.5	0.6–0.9	>0.9
Jet density and contour-CW	soft and parabolic	Dense, variable contour	Dense, triangular with early peaking
Hepatic vein flow	Systolic dominance	Systolic blunting	Systolic reversal

It is extremely important to understand that, as is the cases with all valve regurgitant jets, the severity of the TR jet is not related to the pressure gradient between the RA and RV. It is possible to have severe TR and very low gradient, and to have minimal TR and an extremely high gradient between the two chambers.

The values for mild, moderate, and severe tricuspid regurgitation measurements are shown in Table 6.1. Based on this classification, the treatment plan for tricuspid regurgitation can be determined (Table 6.2).

Tricuspid stenosis

Tricuspid stenosis is another clinical entity that must be ruled out during routine echocardiography. It is a rare condition, but can have many possible etiologies. These include:

• Carcinoid syndrome
• Endocarditis
• Endomyocardial fibrosis
• Lupus Erythematosus
• Congenital malformations.

Tricuspid stenosis gradient severity cutoffs have not been clearly established.

Table 6.2 Tricuspid valve disease surgery indications.	
Class/Indication	Level of evidence
Class I Tricuspid valve repair is beneficial for severe tricuspid regurgitation in patients with MV disease requiring MV surgery.	B
Class IIa Tricuspid valve replacement or annuloplasty is reasonable for severe primary TR when symptomatic.	C
Tricupsid valve replacement is reasonable for severe TR secondary to diseased/abnormal tricuspid valve leaflets not amendable to annuloplasty or repair.	C
Class IIb Tricuspid annuloplasty may be considered for less than severe TR in patients undergoing MV surgery when there is pulmonary hypertension or tricuspid annular dilatation.	C
Class III Tricuspid valve replacement or annuloplasty is not indicated in asymptomatic patients with TR whole pulmonary artery systolic pressure is < 60 mm Hg in the presence of a normal MV.	C
Tricuspid valve replacement or annuloplasty is not indicated in patients with mild primary TR.	C

- Normal gradient is less than 2 mm Hg while the patient is in expiration.
- Severe stenosis is considered when gradient is more than 7 mm Hg.
- Any pressure half-time value of tricuspid valve inflow of 190 ms or less is indicative of severe stenosis.

All measurements of tricuspid stenosis which suggest a diagnosis of hemodynamically significant stenosis are shown in Table 6.3.

Another extremely important piece of information that is obtained from echocardiography of the tricuspid valve is the estimation of RV systolic function. This information is obtained by obtaining the Tricuspid Annular Plane Systolic Excursion (TAPSE) [2, 3].

To obtain TAPSE (Figure 6.9):

1 Obtain a good image of the tricuspid valve in the apical four-chamber view (Figure 6.9a).
2 Place M-mode (dashed line) cursor through the anterior leaflet of the tricuspid valve (Figure 6.9b).
3 Start M-mode imaging (Figure 6.9c).

Table 6.3 Tricuspid stenosis: findings indicative of hemodynamic stenosis.

Specific findings	
Mean pressure gradient (mm Hg)	≥5
Inflow time-velocity integral (cm)	>60
$T_{1/2}$ (ms)	≥190
Valve area by continuity equation (cm²)	≤1
Supportive findings	
Enlarged right atrium ≥ moderate	
Dilated inferior vena cava	

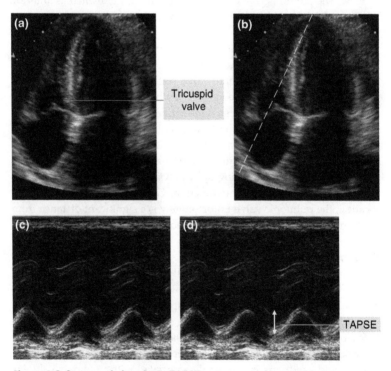

Figure 6.9 Steps needed to obtain TAPSE.

4 Measure the distance the leaflet travels from its lowest position on the M-mode image in diastole, to its highest position on the M-mode in systole.

5 That vertical distance is the TAPSE (Figure 6.9d).

Studies have clear shown that a TAPSE value of < 1.8 cm is associated with greater RV systolic dysfunction and worse outcomes.

Pulmonic valve

- The pulmonic valve is a trileaflet structure that divides the right ventricular outflow tract from the main pulmonary artery.
- A normal pulmonic valve allows for near laminar blood flow during systole from the right ventricle to the pulmonary artery, and has minimal regurgitant flow during diastole.
- The pulmonic valve is the most difficult of the four cardiac valves to visualize on the transthoracic echocardiogram.
- The pulmonic valve is typically only viewed from the parasternal location, and typically only one or two leaflets can be seen in any single view. The pulmonic valve leaflets are anatomically named as anterior, right, and left, with the anterior cusp analogous to the noncoronary cusp of the aortic valve.
- As in other valves, M-mode, color and spectral Doppler images across the pulmonic valve can be obtained.
- By convention, the pulmonic valve leaflets are not typically named individually, but rather the valve as a whole is described as normal or abnormal along with the lesion indentified.
- The short axis plane of the pulmonic valve is normally oriented at 90° from the short axis of the aortic valve. If both valves are visualized in short axis in the same image, transposition of the great vessels should be suspected.

Transesophageal echocardiography plays a modest role in determining pulmonic valve structure and function. Given its anterior anatomical location, the pulmonic valve unfortunately is a significant distance from the transesophageal transducer and is not easily visualized.

Pulmonic stenosis
- Isolated pulmonic stenosis is typically a congenital lesion characterized by fusion of the valve leaflets with resulting decrease in valve area. Anatomically, the leaflets may appear very mobile but they have typical "doming" during systole.
- Rheumatic pulmonic stenosis is rare and almost never occurs without associated left sided valvular involvement.
- Carcinoid syndrome is commonly associated with pulmonic valvular destruction resulting in various degrees of pulmonic valve stenosis and regurgitation. Additionally, the presence of a ventricular septal defect, subpulmonic membrane, or hypertrophic cardiomyopathy may lead to infundibular stenosis within the right ventricular outflow tract itself.

Evaluation of the stenotic pulmonic valve is similar to evaluation of a stenotic aortic valve except that pulmonic valve areas are rarely calculated.

The determination of pulmonic valve stenosis severity is accomplished primarily by determining the pressure gradient:
- Parasternal short axis view of the base is used (Figure 6.10).
- Valve morphology can be assessed in this view. Careful attention should be made to identify calcifications, dysplasia, and a classic domed appearance of the valve.
- Continuous wave Doppler line (dashed line) is then aligned with the right ventricular outflow tract through the pulmonic valve and peak transpulmonic velocity is obtained (Figure 6.11).

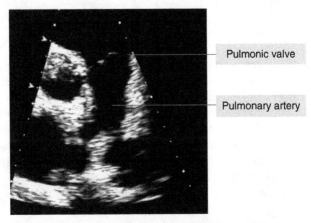

Pulmonic valve

Pulmonary artery

Figure 6.10 PSAX view of the base; the pulmonary artery and pulmonic valve are seen in this view.

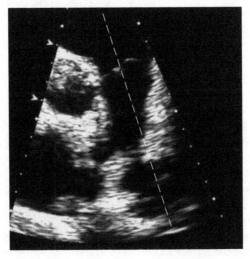

Figure 6.11 Alignment of Doppler to record pulmonic valve VTI in PSAX view of the base.

Table 6.4 Pulmonic stenosis severity by Doppler.

	Mild	Moderate	Severe
Peak velocity (m/s)	<3	3–4	>4
Peak gradient (mmHg)	<36	36–64	>64

- The severity of pulmonic valve stenosis can then be determined from this velocity (Table 6.4 [4]).

Pulmonic regurgitation

Varying degrees of pulmonic regurgitation are quite prevalent in the general population with up to 75% of normal subjects exhibiting either trace or mild pulmonic regurgitation [5]. These small amounts are typically without consequence and can be considered a normal incidental finding when the remainder of the echocardiogram is normal. More significant degrees of pulmonic regurgitation are associated with increasing pulmonary hypertension and/or right ventricular abnormalities. As with pulmonic stenosis, the valve leaflets should be carefully inspected for abnormalities including perforation and vegetations (Table 6.5).

- Pulmonic regurgitation is visualized from a transthoracic parasternal short axis through the base of the heart.
- Color Doppler is applied over the region of the pulmonic valve and regurgitant flow can be visualized returning to the RVOT from the main pulmonary artery.
- The degree of pulmonic regurgitation can be qualitatively appreciated based on the width of the regurgitant jet.
- Other clues to the severity of pulmonic regurgitation are the presence of a dilated right ventricle, with increased right ventricular end diastolic diameter correlating with increasing severity of pulmonic regurgitation, and increased forward RVOT stroke volume relative to aortic stroke volume.

The CW pulmonic regurgitation jet provides clues for severity of regurgitation:

- A denser Doppler envelope represents higher degrees of pulmonic regurgitation.
- Rate of flow deceleration can be determined and used to assess the degree of pulmonic regurgitation. Analogous to aortic regurgitation, a shorter deceleration time, or more rapid pressure decline is indicative of more severe valvular regurgitation. In contrast to aortic regurgitation, there is limited data to correlate specific values with regurgitant severity, but rather a qualitative approach is typically used.

Table 6.5 Indications for balloon valvotomy in pulmonic stenosis.

Class/Indication	Level of evidence
Class I Balloon valvotomy is recommended in adolescent and young adult patients with pulmonic stenosis who have exertional dyspnea, angina, syncope, or presyncope and an RV-to-pulmonary artery peak-to-peak gradient greater than 30 mm Hg at catheterization.	C
Balloon valvotomy is recommended in asymptomatic adolescent and young adult patients with pulmonic stenosis and RV-to-pulmonary artery peak-to-peak gradient greater than 40 mm Hg at catheterization.	C
Class IIb Balloon valvotomy may be reasonable in asymptomatic adolescent and young adult patients with pulmonic stenosis and an RV-to-pulmonary artery peak-to-peak gradient 30–39 mm Hg at catheterization.	C
Class III Balloon valvotomy is not recommended in asymptomatic adolescent and young adult patients with pulmonic stenosis and RV-to-pulmonary artery peak-to-peak gradient <30 mm Hg at catheterization.	C

Further Doppler measurements can be obtained from the pulmonic valve regurgitant jet to determine pulmonary vascular hemodynamic parameters. Most important of these measurements is the measurement of the pulmonary end diastolic velocity:

- The pulmonary regurgitation jet is visualized in the parasternal short axis view of the base or the RV outflow view (Figure 6.12).
- In color Doppler, the PI jet is sometimes described as having appearance of a "flame". A PW, or CW, through the regurgitation jet is recorded (Figure 6.13).
- The point of interest is at the end of the regurgitant flow, before the flow ceases. To calculate the pulmonary artery end diastolic pressure, this value is plugged into the equation:

$$PAEDP = 4 \times PAEDV^2 + RAP$$

- This value has been shown to correlate well with the pulmonary capillary wedge pressure and may give information regarding left sided filling pressures.

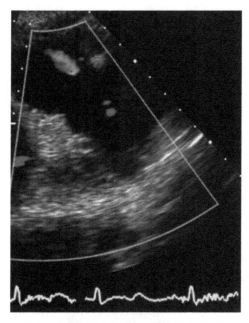

Figure 6.12 Visualization of PI jet using color Doppler in the PSAX view of the base.

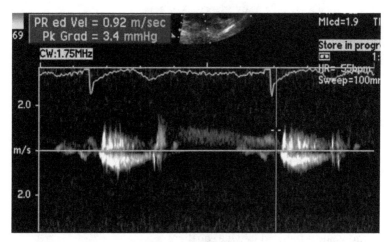

Figure 6.13 PW Doppler of PI jet. The point marked on the image is used to measure the PADP.

For a comprehensive review of the indications and guidelines for management of valvular heart disease, the ACC/AHA guidelines initially published in 2006 and updated in 2008 should be referred to [6, 7].

Box 6.1 Step-by-step guide to calculating the Q_p/Q_s ratio

Q_P/Q_S = Pulmonary flow / Systemic flow
      (usually done via RVOT VTI / LVOT VTI)

Step 1: In a parasternal short axis view at the base, identify the RVOT. Measure the diameter of the RVOT.
Step 2: Record the CW Dopppler at the level of the RVOT. Record the RVOT VTI in systole
Step 3: In parasternal long axis view, zoom in on the LVOT. Measure the diameter of the LVOT.
Step 4: In apical view, record the PW Doppler at the level of the LVOT. Record LVOT VTI in systole.

Note that other valves can be used to calculate the $Q_p/_Q$s, as long as the anatomic location used is distal to the location of the intracardiac shunt.

Q_p/Q_s: Pulmonary to systemic flow ratio

- Is used when shunt is suspected or diagnosed.
- Can be determined using echocardiography.
- Good views of left sided and right sided structures are essential for an accurate calculation.
- A step-by-step guide to determining Q_p/Q_s is shown in Box 6.1.
- Cutoff for intervention is a shunt ratio of at least 2:1, although the clinical presentation is extremely important in deciding whether to intervene on a shunt.

References

1 Anwar AM, Geleijnse ML, Soliman OII, *et al.* Assessment of normal tricuspid valve anatomy in adults by real-time three-dimensional echocardiography. *Int J Cardiovasc Imaging* 2007; 23(6):717–24.
2 Tamborini G, Pepi M, Galli CA, *et al.* Feasibility and accuracy of a routine echocardiographic assessment of right ventricular function. *Int J Cardiol* 2007; 115(1)86–9.
3 Kjaergaard J, Akkan D, Iversen KK, *et al.* Right ventricular dysfunction as an independent predictor of short- and long-term mortality in patients with heart failure. *Eur J Heart Fail* 2007; 9(6–7):610–6.
4 Baumgartner H, Hung J, Bermejo J, *et al.* Echocardiographic assessment of valve stenosis: EAE/ASE recommendations for clinical practice. *J Am Soc Echocardiogr* 2009; 22(1):101–2.
5 Zoghbi *et al.* Recommendations for evaluation of the severity of native valvular regurgitation with two-dimensional and Doppler echocardiography. *J Am Soc Echocardiogr* 2003; 16:777–802.

6 Bonow RO, Carabello BA, Kanu C, *et al*. ACC/AHA 2006 Guidelines for the management of patients with valvular heart disease. *Circulation* 2006; 114; 450–527.

7 Bonow RO, Carabello BA, Chatterjee K, *et al*. 2008 Focused update incorporated into the ACC/AHA 2006 guidelines for the management of patients with valvular heart disease. *J Am Coll Cardiol* 2008; 52(13):1–142.

Prosthetic heart valves

Karthik Gujja[1] and Vladimir Fridman[2]

[1]Division of Cardiology, Department of Internal Medicine, Long Island College Hospital, New York, USA
[2]Cardiovascular Diseases, New York, NY, USA

CHAPTER 7

Prosthetic heart valves add another level of complexity to the performance of an echocardiogram. There are multiple different types and multiple different echocardiographic signatures of prosthetic valves. Furthermore, many forms of prosthetic valve malfunction exist, and in some cases these are life threatening and must be diagnosed immediately.

The types of prosthetic valves/valve repairs are:

- mechanical valves
- tissue (biological) valves
- valved conduits
- annular rings.

There are multiple mechanical valves available on the market. Some of the most common types and their characteristics are:

- Bileaflet tilting disc valves
  - two pyrolytic carbon semicircular discs attached to a rigid valve ring by small hinges;
  - opening angle 75–90°;
  - three orifices: one small central and two larger lateral orifices;
  - Normal regurgitant volume of 5–10 ml.
- Single tilting disc valves
  - circular sewing ring;
  - circular disc eccentrically attached by metal struts;
  - opening angle 60–80°;
  - flow occurs through major and minor orifices.
- Ball-in-cage valve
  - circular sewing ring;
  - silastic or metal ball;

Practical Manual of Echocardiography in the Urgent Setting, First Edition.
Edited by Vladimir Fridman and Mario J. Garcia.
© 2013 John Wiley & Sons, Ltd. Published 2013 by John Wiley & Sons, Ltd.

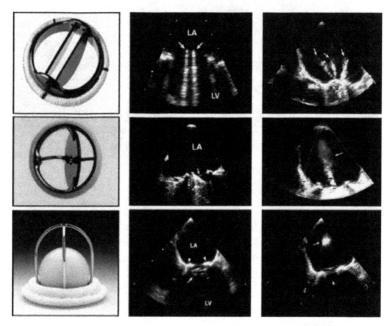

Figure 7.1 Mechanical valves and their echocardiographic images with normal regurgitation profiles: top – bileaflet; middle – single leaflet; bottom – ball and cage valves (Reproduced from [1], with permission from Elsevier).

    ○ cage with arches;
    ○ high profile;
    ○ flow occurs around the ball;
    ○ normal regurgitant volume of 2–5 ml.

The common mechanical prosthetic valves, and their normal regurgitation profiles, are shown in Figure 7.1.

There are multiple types of tissue valves as well. Some basic characteristics are:

- Stented heterograft valves
    ○ sewing ring with three semirigid stents or struts;
    ○ trileaflet – opens to a circular orifice;
    ○ suboptimal hemodynamic profile compared to native valves;
    ○ normal regurgitant volume of about 1 ml;
    ○ 10% exhibit a small degree of regurgitation by color flow imaging.
- Stentless heterograft valves
    ○ manufactured from intact animal aortic valves;
    ○ usually in the aortic position;
    ○ no rigid stents present – larger effective orifice area;
    ○ better hemodynamic profile compared to stented biological valves.

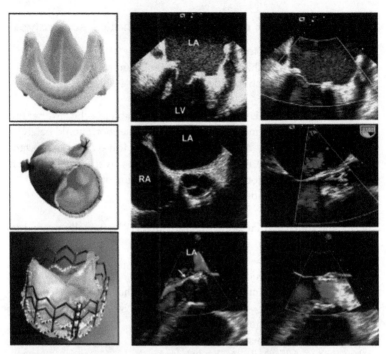

Figure 7.2 Common bioprosthetic valves and their echocardiographic features in diastole (middle) and systole (right): top – stented; middle – stentless; bottom – percutaneous valves (Reproduced from [1], with permission from Elsevier).

- Homograft valves
  - antibiotic-sterilized, cryogenically preserved, valves harvested from human cadavers;
  - favorable hemodynamics, resistant to infection, no anticoagulation requirement;
  - usually implanted as a complete root replacement with coronary artery reimplantation.
- Autograft valves (Ross procedure)
  - native pulmonary valve replaces the diseased aortic valve (the native pulmonary valve is thus the autograft);
  - stentless homograft is placed in the pulmonary position;
- Percutaneous valves
  - recently, valve replacements – pulmonic and aortic valves – have been done percutaneously via transapical or transfemoral approaches;
  - imaging and hemodynamic characteristics are similar to those of stentless biological valves.

Some common bioprosthetic valves and their echocardiographic features are shown in Figure 7.2.

Echocardiographic approach to prosthetic heart valves

- Evaluation is similar to that of native valves.
- Reverberations and shadowing play a significant role.
- Fluid dynamics of each specific valve prosthesis influences the Doppler findings.

For all valve types, it is important to do a complete echocardiogram, including all necessary measurements. Careful attention should be given to all the hemodynamics of any prosthetic valve. However, it is important to note that just because a patient has a prosthetic valve, it does not mean that their clinical situation is due to the malfunction of the valve.

Echo measurements for all prosthetic valves [1]:

1 Complete 2D imaging, all standard views.
2 Calculate transvalvular pressure gradient – CW is usually needed to prevent aliasing.
3 Calculate valve orifice area
   - dependent on location of valve;
   - similar to measurements of native valve in the respective position;
   - can use:
     ○ continuity equation;
     ○ pressure half time;
     ○ dimensionless index (velocity based).
4 Estimate degree of regurgitation.
5 Check if the regurgitation occurs within the contours of the valve, or outside of the valve (paravalvular leak).
6 Assess ventricular size and function.
7 If any post-valve replacement echo study exists, the current results MUST be compared to that study to check for any changes in hemodynamics/structures.

Normal echocardiographic appearance of prosthetic valves includes [1]:

- Tissue valves
  ○ stented valves – three cusps and struts with echogenic sewing ring;
  ○ stentless valves – thickening of aortic root/annulus, as usually in aortic position;
  ○ homograft/autograft – increased echogenicity at the annular level.
- Mechanical valves
  ○ ball-in-cage:
    ■ highly echogenic;
    ■ motion of ball is visible;
  ○ single tilting disc – a single disc is seen moving with systole and diastole;

Table 7.1 Prosthetic aortic valve Doppler parameters (Reproduced from [1], with permission from Elsevier).

Parameter	Normal	Possible stenosis	Suggests significant stenosis
Peak velocity (m/s)	<3	3–4	>4
Mean gradient (mm Hg)	<20	20–35	>35
DVI	≥0.30	0.29–0.25	<0.25
EOA (cm²)	>1.2	1.2–0.8	<0.8
Contour of the jet velocity through the PrAV	Triangular, early peaking	Triangular to intermediate	Rounded, symmetrical contour
AT (ms)	<80	80–100	>100

Table 7.2 Prosthetic mitral valve Doppler parameters (Reproduced from [1], with permission from Elsevier).

	Normal	Possible stenosis	Suggest significant stenosis
Peak velocity (m/s)	<1.9	1.9–2.5	≥2.5
Mean gradient (mm Hg)	≤5	6–10	>10
VTI_{PrMV}/VTI_{LVO}	<2.2	2.2–2.5	>2.5
EOA (cm²)	≥2.0	1–2	<1
PHT (ms)	<130	130–200	>200

- o bileaflet tilting disc – hemi discs seen moving with systole and diastole (with reverberation of both discs producing a classic appearance).
- Normal hemodynamic measurements (gradients across the valve, areas) are different for all valves, and are easily obtained online.

However, a quick reference guide for detection of prosthetic aortic valve malfunction is shown in Table 7.1.

A quick reference guide for detection of prosthetic mitral valve malfunction is shown in Table 7.2.

There are many reasons for a prosthetic valve to malfunction. Some of the common reasons are:
- structural valve failure
- thrombosis of the valve
- pannus formation
- endocarditis (infection or noninfective)
- stenosis
- regurgitation (valvular or para-valvular)
- patient–prosthesis mismatch.

Approach to suspected valve dysfunction

- TTE.
- If unclear on TTE, TEE is required
  - Mitral valve prosthesis is usually difficult to analyze using TTE due to severe shadowing (especially of the left atrium in the parasternal and apical views), thus a TEE is usually required.
  - Aortic valve prosthesis evaluation is usually adequate with a TTE, if good views are obtained. However, a TEE might still be necessary to further elucidate any problems with the valve.
  - Right-sided valves are usually difficult to fully visualize on a TTE, and a TEE might be required.

Structural valve failure
- Mechanical valves
  - Starr–Edwards silastic valve can have problems with the structural deformation of the ball;
  - Bjork–Shiley valves were single tilting disc valves which were taken off the market due to high numbers of strut failures;
  - breaking off of a disc can lead to disc embolization;
  - tearing, or dislodgment of sutures, can be sometimes visualized;
  - malposition of the annulus of the valve, due to stitch failure or similar problems, can rarely be visualized;
  - structure failure may be intermittent, therefore long recordings are required for proper evaluation.
- Tissue valves
  - failure is much more common than in mechanical valves;
  - calcification, perforation, or spontaneous tissue degeneration of leaflets are the usual causes of failure (Figure 7.3);
  - abnormal regurgitation;
  - usually a gradual process, although it can be acute.

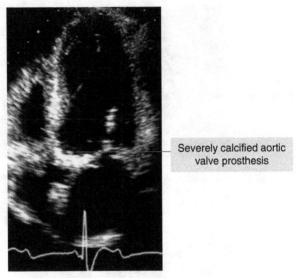

Severely calcified aortic valve prosthesis

Figure 7.3 Severe calcification of a bioprosthetic aortic valve. Gradient measurements indicated the presence of severe aortic stenosis.

Thrombosis (Figure 7.4)
- Almost exclusive of mechanical valves (anticoagulation is always needed with mechanical valves).
- Highest risk: mitral and tricuspid positions.
- Usually associated with inadequate anticoagulation (or if vitamin K is used to reverse anticoagulation for any reason).
- Peripheral embolization of thrombus can be present.
- Hemodynamics are usually consistent with valve stenosis.
- TEE is often needed, especially in the mitral position.

Pannus formation
- Formation of granulation tissue as a result of healing.
- Can encroach on opening of a prosthetic valve, and create a stenosis physiology.
- Minimum is 12 months post-surgery; most common is five years post-surgery.
- More common in mitral valve position than aortic valve position.

Thrombus versus pannus
- The incidence of prosthetic valve obstruction is estimated to be 4% per year [2].

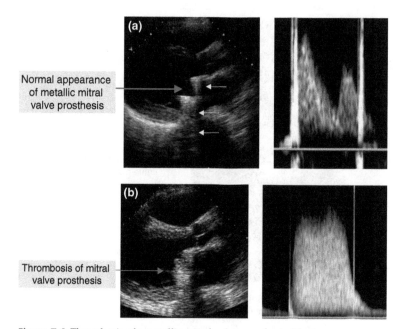

Normal appearance of metallic mitral valve prosthesis

Thrombosis of mitral valve prosthesis

Figure 7.4 Thrombosis of a metallic mitral valve prosthesis. The two echocardiograms were taken from the same patient one month apart. **(a)** A normal appearing metallic valve prosthesis with reverberation artifact (yellow arrows) and a normal CW Doppler inflow profile. **(b)** The mitral valve prosthesis is noted to be thrombosed with a CW Doppler inflow profile consistent with severe valve stenosis.

- Pure thrombus: 75% of cases.
- Pure pannus: 10% of cases.
- Mixed thrombus and pannus: 12%.
- Recent history of embolic event is associated with thrombus/fibrinous structure.
- Thrombi are generally larger and have a density similar to the myocardium.
- Pannus formation usually involves small dense masses that may not be visualized in up to 30% of cases.

Endocarditis (Figures 7.5 and 7.6)
- Approximate risk: 0.5% per year.
- Mechanical valves: vegetation usually on sewing ring.
- Tissue valves: vegetation usually on leaflets.
- Is discussed in detail in later chapters.

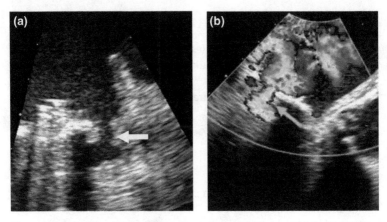

Figure 7.5 Infection of a bileaflet mechanical mitral valve prosthesis resulted in (a) the detachment of the valve annulus from the myocardium (yellow arrow) (b) and severe perivalvular regurgitation.

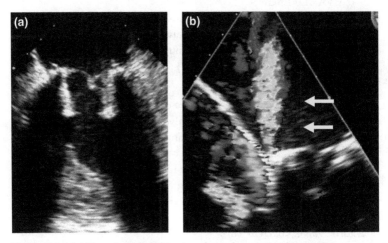

Figure 7.6 (a) Although 2D TEE imaging showed no major abnormalities with a stented bioprosthetic valve in a patient suspected of having endocarditis, (b) color Doppler showed moderate to severe perivalvular regurgitation (yellow arrows) which raises the suspicion for infection of the prosthetic valve.

It is important to remember the differential diagnosis of high gradients in prosthetic valves.
- Actual obstruction.
- High cardiac output state:
  - anemia;
  - fever;
  - thyrotoxicosis.

- Significant regurgitation.
- Patient-prosthesis mismatch.
- Pressure recovery phenomenon (especially bileaflet mechanical valves).

To determine which is the correct diagnosis [1]:

1 Compare to baseline study.
2 Use prosthesis/body surface area to calculate if patient–prosthesis mismatch is present.
3 Results favoring stenosis
   - aortic valve:
     ○ peak velocity >4.5 m/s;
     ○ mean gradient >50 mm Hg;
     ○ effective orifice area <0.8 cm²;
     ○ dimensionless index <0.2–0.25.
   - mitral valve:
     ○ increased peak velocity >2 m/s;
     ○ PHT >200 ms;
     ○ MVA <1.0 1.5 cm²;
     ○ E peak >1.9 m/s; VTI_{PMV}/VTI_{LVOT} >2.2; PHT >130 ms.

Of note, high peak prosthetic mitral valve velocity without an elevated PHT likely represents increase flow through the valve, and not prosthetic valve stenosis.

Valve–prosthesis patient mismatch

- This is a condition where the effective orifice area of a prosthetic valve is less than that of a normal native valve for a specific patient. It occurs due to a sizing problem in the operating room, when a valve smaller in diameter rather than an appropriate valve for a patient's body surface area is placed. The condition results in high gradients, even though there is no pathological condition occurring within the prosthetic valve [3, 4].
- For a specific body surface area, the valve–prosthesis patient mismatch occurs if:
   ○ aortic valve: <0.85 cm²/m²;
   ○ mitral valve <1.2 cm²/m².
- The clinical consequences of this condition are similar to those encountered with stenosis of the respective valve.

Pseudo-regurgitation

This occurs in the setting of a mechanical mitral valve prosthesis. LVOT flow is erroneously projected into the LA, mimicking mitral regurgitation, due to the longer transit time of ultrasound in case of the prosthetic valve [5].

Pressure recovery

The fluid dynamics of blood as it passes through openings within the prosthetic valves are slightly different than those of native valves (especially in metallic valves). One major effect of such flow is the increase in flow velocity as it passes through the prosthetic valve orifice. The velocity decreases distal to the valve. However, due to the nature of Doppler signaling, the highest velocity is recorded, and thus a higher than actual transvalvular gradient is obtained [6, 7, 8].

Prosthetic valve regurgitation is another possible source of valve malfunction. In tissue valves, common causes are degenerative changes, infective endocarditis, and paravalvular leak. In mechanical valves, common causes are dehiscence, thrombosis, pannus formation, and infection.

It is important to differentiate between normal and abnormal prosthetic valvular regurgitation [9].

"Normal regurgitation" is usually:
- symmetric
- brief
- nonturbulent
- within the volume limits for specific valves (as stated above)
- does not increase velocity or gradients.

Abnormal regurgitation is usually:
- asymmetric
- of long duration
- turbulent
- causes hemodynamic changes such as pulmonary HTN (in case of mitral valve).

As in native valve regurgitation, a thorough TTE, and sometimes TEE, is necessary to fully define the nature, volume, and cause of valvular regurgitation (Figure 7.7).

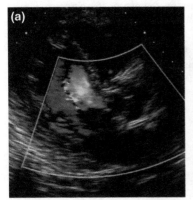 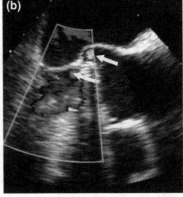

Figure 7.7 (a) A TTE in a patient with shortness of breath showed the presence of a metallic aortic valve prosthesis with moderate aortic insufficiency. (b) A follow-up TEE demonstrated that the aortic regurgitation was perivalvular (yellow arrows) in origin.

It is true that the presence of a prosthetic valve, or valves, makes performing and interpreting an echocardiogram more complex. However, analyzing the valve from all possible views, and recording all of the appropriate measurements for each prosthetic valve will make drawing conclusions about the function of such a valve easier and more accurate.

References

1 Zoghbi WA, Chambers JB, Dumesnil JG, *et al*. Recommendations for Evaluation of Prosthetic Valves with Echocardiography and Doppler Ultrasound. *J Am Soc Echocardiogr* 2009; 22(9):975-1014 (doi:10.1016/j.echo.2009.07.013).

2 Vongpatanasin, W, Hillis, LD, Lange, RA. Prosthetic heart valves. *N Engl J Med* 1996; 335:407.

3 Pibarot P, Dumesnil JG. Hemodynamic and clinical impact of prosthesis–patient mismatch in the aortic valve position and its prevention. *J Am Coll Cardiol* 2000; 36; 1131–41.

4 Hanayama N, Christakis GT, Mallidi HR, *et al*. Patient prosthesis mismatch is rare after aortic valve replacement: valve size may be irrelevant. *Ann Thorac Surg* 2002; 73:1822–9.

5 Rudski LG, Chow CM, Levine RA. Prosthetic mitral regurgitation can be mimicked by Doppler color flow mapping: Avoiding misdiagnosis. *J Am Soc Echo* 2004; 17(8):829–33.

6 Baumgartner H, Khan S, DeRobertis M, *et al*. Effect of prosthetic aortic valve design on the Doppler-catheter gradient correlation: an *in vitro* study of normal St. Jude, Medtronic-Hall, Starr-Edwards and Hancock valves. *J Am Coll Cardiol* 1992; 19:324–32.

7 Baumgartner H, Khan S, DeRobertis M, *et al*. Discrepancies between Doppler and catheter gradients in aortic prosthetic valves *in vitro*. A manifestation of localized gradients and pressure recovery. *Circulation* 1990; 82:1467–75.

8 Levin RA, Schwammenthal E. Stenosis in the eye of the observer: impact of pressure recovery on assessing aortic valve area. *J Am Col Cardiol* 2003; 41(3):443–5.

9 Ionescu A, Fraser AG, Butchart EG. Prevalence and clinical significance of incidental paraprosthetic valvular regurgitation: a prospective study using transoesophageal echocardiography. *Heart* 2003; 89:1316–21.

The great vessels

Vladimir Fridman[1] and Hejmadi Prabhu[2]
[1]Cardiovascular Diseases, New York, NY, USA
[2]Cardiovascular Diseases, Wyckoff Heights Medical Center,
New York, NY, USA

CHAPTER 8

Every echocardiogram must provide the visualization of, and some basic information, about the great vessels. This includes the ascending and, in some views, the descending aorta and the proximal portion of the pulmonary artery. The information about the great vessels can in many cases be extremely important to the diagnosis and management of acute cardiovascular syndromes.

Aorta

The proximal ascending aorta, as well as small portions of the descending and abdominal aorta, can be visualized on routine echocardiography. The views involved are:

- Parasternal long axis view (Figure 8.1)
  - the best source of measurement of the diameter of the ascending aorta;
  - points of measurement are:
    - aortic valve annulus (white dotted line);
    - sinuses of Valsalva (yellow dotted line);
    - sinotubular junction (green dotted line);
    - ascending aorta distal to the junction (blue dotted line);
    - the descending thoracic aorta is also visualized in this view posterior to the heart (blue arrow).
- Apical five-chamber view
  - provides a good view of the proximal portion of the ascending aorta.
- Apical three-chamber view
  - able to visualize a large portion of the ascending aorta.

Practical Manual of Echocardiography in the Urgent Setting, First Edition.
Edited by Vladimir Fridman and Mario J. Garcia.
© 2013 John Wiley & Sons, Ltd. Published 2013 by John Wiley & Sons, Ltd.

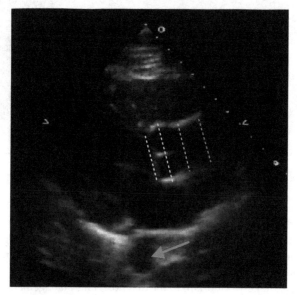

Figure 8.1 Parasternal long axis view of the aorta; various structures are noted, as described in the text.

- Suprasternal view
  - ○ excellent view to look for the aortic arch and the vessels coming off of it (brachiocephalic artery, L common carotid artery, L subclavian artery);
  - ○ difficult to obtain and usually requires advanced experience in performing echocardiography.
- Subcostal view
  - ○ with manipulation, the abdominal portion of the descending aorta can be visualized close to the liver;
  - ○ it is difficult to differentiate abdominal aorta from the IVC and/or hepatic vein in many cases;
  - ○ color Doppler or PW Doppler showing pulsatile flow, in the appropriate direction, can prove that the aorta is in the field of view.

Aortic emergency

There are four main aortic emergencies. These are:

1 aortic dissection
2 intramural hematoma
3 penetrating aortic ulcer
4 traumatic or iatrogenic dissection/transection.

Although the gold standard imaging modality for these emergencies are CT and/or MRI, many times the patients who have such presentations are unstable and an echocardiogram, especially a TEE, is the diagnostic modality of choice. It is, therefore, extremely important to know about these emergent conditions, and to know how to diagnose them using echocardiography.

Aortic dissection [1]

It is extremely important not only to diagnose an aortic dissection, but to also determine whether it starts proximal to or distal to the left subclavian artery (Stanford type A and B, respectively).

- an intimal flap is sometimes directly visualized using TTE or TEE;
- a TTE is useful in diagnosing a dissection in the proximal aortic arch;
- a TEE is useful in diagnosing a dissection in the ascending aorta, aortic arch, and proximal descending aorta;
- color Doppler can be used to determine:
  - whether two separate flow patterns exist within the aorta, indicating a dissection;
  - which is the true lumen – the lumen that has pulsatile flow in the appropriate direction.

It is extremely important to note that a TEE can diagnose an aortic dissection down to the level of the stomach, since the probe does not pass more caudal than that. Therefore, abdominal aortic dissections are extremely hard to diagnose with echocardiography. There is also a TEE "blind spot" in the proximal aortic arch, which is extremely hard to examine due to the attenuation of the ultrasound beam from the trachea/bronchus. To make a diagnosis of aortic dissection, the intimal flap should be seen in more than one view/plane. The sensitivity of TEE to make a diagnosis of aortic dissection is 97%, and specificity is around 80–95%.

In TEE views of the aorta, frequently a mirror artifact appears to mimic an intimal flap and aortic dissection. It is extremely important to differentiate between a true aortic dissection and mirror artifact. In mirror artifact, there appears to be two distinct aortas – one behind the other, and color Doppler shows pulsatile flow in opposite directions. In a true dissection, an intimal flap is usually seen moving within the aorta and color Doppler shows differing blood flow profiles between the true and false lumens.

TTE can demonstrate complications of ascending aortic dissection, including aortic insufficiency, pericardial effusion and cardiac tamponade.

Figure 8.2 shows an aortic dissection as seen on the apical three-chamber view of a TTE. Figure 8.3 shows a short axis view of the aorta with a clearly visible intimal flap (arrow). Figure 8.4 show TEE views of aortic dissection. It has color Doppler imaging showing flow in the true lumen (arrows), while no flow is seen in the false lumen.

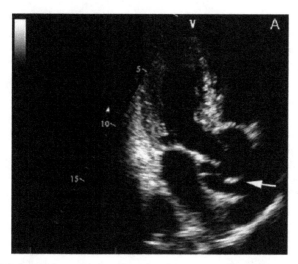

Figure 8.2 Apical three-chamber view showing an intimal flap in the ascending aorta (arrow) (Reproduced from Brunson *et al.* [2], with permission from Elsevier).

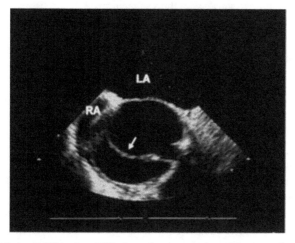

Figure 8.3 Aortic dissection: TEE view of a cross-section of the aorta showing a clearly visible intimal flap (arrow) (Reproduced from Song *et al.* [3], with permission from Elsevier).

Intramural hematoma [1]

- Is classified using the Stanford Classification, as are aortic dissections.
- Involves rupture of the aortic vaso vasorum and bleeding into the aortic media.

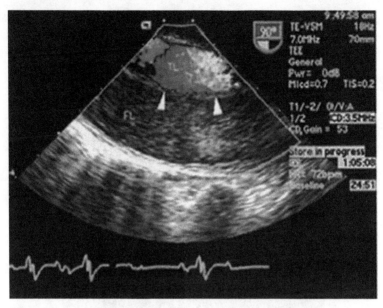

Figure 8.4 Color Doppler of an aortic dissection showing flow in the true lumen (arrowhead) and no flow in the false lumen (FL) (Reproduced from Orsini *et al.* [4], with permission from Elsevier).

- Difficult to diagnose on echocardiography.
- Involves seeing thickening and thrombus within the aortic wall (Figure 8.5).
- TEE, usually by an experienced operator, is required to make the correct diagnosis.

Penetrating aortic ulcer [1]
- Involves ulceration of atheromatous plaque with rupture of the internal elastic lamina and hematoma formation in the media (Figure 8.6).
- Rarely occurs in the proximal aorta; mainly occurs in the distal thoracic aorta.
- A TEE is required if diagnosis is to be made via echocardiography.
- To make the diagnosis, an ulcer is visualized within the aortic wall.

Traumatic or iatrogenic dissection [6]
- Should be suspected in any appropriate clinical situation.
- Involves direct physical damage to the aorta, whether from trauma or any invasive medical intervention.
- The most dangerous clinical situation in this category is an aortic transection, in which the aorta is either torn or ruptured.

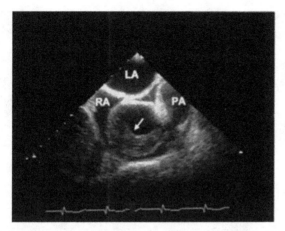

Figure 8.5 Intramural hematoma: a cross-section of the aorta shows thickening of the aortic wall (arrow), which is a classic finding of an intramural hematoma (Reproduced from Song *et al.* [3], with permission from Elsevier).

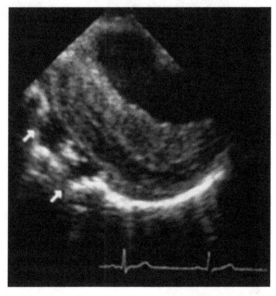

Figure 8.6 Multiple penetrating aortic ulcers are noted (arrows) as well as thrombus within the aortic wall (Reproduced from Vilacosta *et al.* [5], with permission from Elsevier).

Besides emergent situations, there are multiple other aortic diseases that can be diagnosed by echocardiography.

• Aortic aneurysm – the size of all the visualized segments of the aorta can, and should be, recorded. Any dilatation should be followed clinically, based on the current aortic disease guidelines.

- Aortic atheromas
  - need to be assessed when TEE is done for CVA/TIA/embolic reasons;
  - plaques within the walls are clearly visible as echo-dense structures within the aortic wall on TEE;
  - plaque size should be recorded;
  - if large plaques (usually a diameter of 0.4 cm is the cutoff for a large atheroma), antiplatelet and/or anticoagulation therapy should be considered for the patient as per guidelines.
- Aortic coarctation
  - a congenital condition where the aorta narrows in the area of ligamentum arteriosum;
  - can cause high blood pressure in the upper extremities with normal/low blood pressure in the lower extremities;
  - can be diagnosed via a TTE (suprasternal view) or TEE;
  - characterized by increased velocities on CW Doppler and turbulence on Color Doppler in the appropriate anatomical location;
  - characteristic CW Doppler pattern shows high velocity systolic flow (showing the gradient between areas proximal to and distal to the coarctation via Gradient = $4V^2$) and small velocity holodiastolic flow due to an existent diastolic gradient between the areas proximal to and distal to the coarctation;
  - CT and/or MR are the gold standard for diagnosis and are needed to guide treatment in this condition.

Pulmonary artery

The pulmonary artery is an important vessel to visualize during echocardiography for multiple reasons. However, the main problem with imaging this artery is the inability of both TTE and TEE to provide clear views of the vessel. The views that can be attempted to image the pulmonary artery are:
- with TTE:
  - RV outflow view – can see the main pulmonary artery and the bifurcation into the right and left pulmonary arteries;
  - PSAX at the base – can see the pulmonic valve and the pulmonary artery as well as possible view of the pulmonary artery bifurcation;
  - suprasternal view – the right pulmonary artery is seen with its usual relation to the aorta (if one is in cross-section, the other one must be longitudinal if there is no anatomical defect present).
- with TEE:
  - It is best visualized in the mid esophageal right ventricular inflow outflow, upper esophageal aortic arch short axis, and midesophageal ascending aortic short axis views. In these views, the pulmonary

artery with the bifurcation into the right and left pulmonary arteries are clearly visualized. Again, the right pulmonary artery is seen with its close anatomical relationship to the aorta.

The reasons for attempting to visualize the pulmonary artery are:

- Pulmonary embolus
    - likely the most important indication to imaging the pulmonary artery;
    - the diameter of the PA artery should be recorded in any such case (more details are given in later chapters);
    - rarely an actual thrombus can be seen either in the pulmonary artery or in one of the main branches of the pulmonary artery (Figure 8.7).
- Pulmonary HTN – although measuring of pulmonary artery systolic pressures by echocardiography does not require direct visualization of the pulmonary artery, a dilated pulmonary artery is associated with pulmonary hypertension.
- Evidence of a left to right shunt on a color Doppler imaging of the pulmonary artery, and the systolic and diastolic flow through the shunt should point to the operator to the diagnosis of a PDA if the flow is located in the correct anatomical location.
- Other congenital abnormalities – the determination of relationships of the great vessels to other cardiac structures is extremely important in diagnosing congenital cardiac abnormalities.

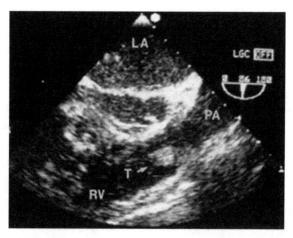

Figure 8.7 A TEE view showing a thrombus (T) located in the right ventricle (RV) migrating toward the pulmonary artery (PA) (Reproduced from Van Der Wouw *et al.* [7], with permission from Elsevier).

- Pulmonic stenosis – to record the gradient across the pulmonic valve via CW Doppler, a clear view showing the RVOT, pulmonic valve, and the proximal portion of the pulmonary artery should be obtained.

Pulmonary artery pressure measurement

Pulmonary arterial hypertension is a complicated clinical disorder. There are multiple different etiologies for this condition and different treatments. However, the most important role of echocardiography is establishing the pulmonary artery systolic and diastolic pressures. Although the gold standard measurement is a right heart catheterization, this is simply too invasive for a screening test. As such, the most commonly used test to check pulmonary artery pressure is an echocardiogram.

On echocardiography, the three measurements that can be obtained are:
1 Pulmonary artery systolic pressure.
2 Pulmonary artery diastolic pressure.
3 Mean pulmonary artery pressure.

Pulmonary artery systolic pressure
- Derived via tricuspid regurgitation jet.
- A CW Doppler through the tricuspid regurgitation jet is recorded.
- Peak regurgitant velocity (v) is recorded.
- Pressure gradient between RV and RA $= 4v^2$
- RA pressure + pressure gradient = PASP
- RA pressure is taken via measurement of IVC (in subcostal view), as described in Chapter 4.

Pulmonary artery diastolic pressure (PADP)
- Derived via the pulmonary regurgitation jet.
- CW (or PW) of pulmonary artery regurgitation jet is recorded in the parasternal short axis view of the base (Figure 8.8).
- The velocity (v) of the jet at the final point of regurgitation (end diastole) is recorded (Figure 8.8).
- The pressure gradient between PA and RV in diastole $= 4v^2$
- To this number, we add the RAP (as described in Chapter 4), and this sum is equal to the pulmonary artery diastolic pressure.

Mean pulmonary artery pressure (MPAP)
- MPAP can be estimated from the pulmonary artery acceleration time.
- CW Doppler is taken of the pulmonic valve in the parasternal short axis view at the base.
- The characteristic flow profile appears in Figure 8.9.
- The time from begining of flow into the pulmonary artery to the point where flow reaches peak velocity is measured, as shown in Figure 8.9.
- MPAP = 79 – 0.45(acceleration time in milliseconds).

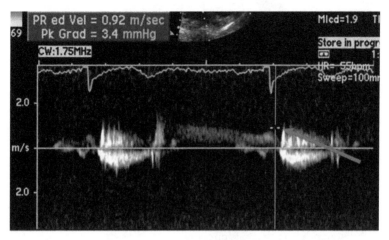

Figure 8.8 Measuring the pulmonary artery diastolic pressure. The CW Doppler of the pulmonary regurgitation jet is seen above the baseline flow in diastole. The end point of diastole (arrow) is the point of interest, the gradient corresponding to which is the gradient between end diastolic RV and PA pressure.

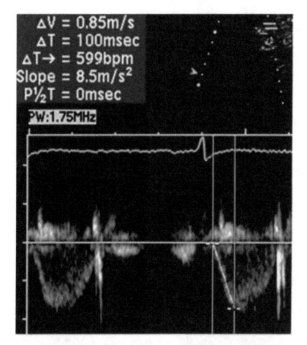

Figure 8.9 Profile of pulmonic flow. The time from the start of pulmonic flow to the peak velocity of flow is measured, 100 ms in this case, to determine the mean pulmonary artery pressure (Reproduced from Mahan *et al.* [8], with permission from Lippincott Williams & Wilkins).

D-septal shift

One notable feature of elevated right-sided pressures is interventricular septal flattening. Either in systole, diastole, or both, in this condition interventricular septum bows toward the left ventricle. This makes the LV in the parasternal short axis view resemble the letter "D", as opposed to its usual ovoid shape (Figure 8.10).

If the D-septal shift happens in systole, it is indicative of right-sided pressure overload, in diastole it is indicative of right-sided volume overload.

It is important to pay attention to the presence of the "D" Sign, as it can give a lot of clues to the hemodynamics of the patient without a need for complex calculations. This is especially important for echos that are performed in "difficult"patients (usually ICU, severe COPD, vented patients), where full hemodynamic calculations are difficult.

Overall, imaging of the great vessels using echocardiography is complex, but extremely important. In many clinical situations, echocardiography and visualization of the great vessels can establish the diagnosis of life-threatening conditions and can significantly reduce the time to initiation of treatment for these patients. However, imaging the great

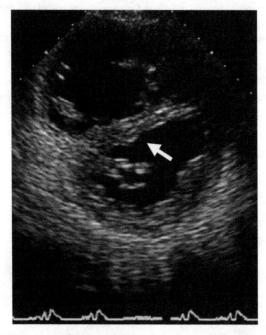

Figure 8.10 Interventricular septal (arrow) flattening noted in diastole, indicating right-sided volume overload.

vessels by echocardiography is difficult and, as always, an experienced echocardiographer should be available to interpret the images, especially when attempting to diagnose life-threatening conditions in unstable patients.

References

1 Lansman SL, Saunders PC, Malekan R, Spielvogel D. Acute aortic syndrome. *J Thorac Cardiovasc Surg* 2010; 140(6):S92–7.
2 Brunson JM, Fine RL, Schussler JM. Acute ascending aortic dissection diagnosed with transthoracic echocardiography. *J Am Soc Echocardiogr* 2009; 22(9): 1086e5–7.
3 Song JK, Kim HS, Kang DH, *et al*. Different clinical features of aortic intramural hematoma versus dissection involving the ascending aorta. *J Am Coll Cardiol* 2001; 37(6):1604–10.
4 Orsini AN, Kolias TJ, Strelich KR, *et al*. Feasibility of transesophageal echocardiography with a ten-french monoplane probe. *J Am Soc Echocardiogr* 2003; 16(6):682–7.
5 Vilacosta I, San Roman JA, Aragoncillo P, *et al*. Penetrating atherosclerotic aortic ulcer: documentation by transesophageal echocardiography. *J Am Coll Cardiol* 1998; 32(1):83–9.
6 Marcura KJ, Corl FM, Fishman EK, Bluemke DA. Pathogenesis in acute aortic syndromes: aortic aneurysm leak and rupture and traumatic aortic transection. *Am J Roentg* 2003; 181(2):303–307.
7 Van Der Wouw, PA, Koster RW, Delemarre BJ, *et al*. Diagnostic accuracy of transesophageal echocardiography during cardiopulmonary resuscitation. *J Am Coll Cardiol* 1997; 30(3):780–3.
8 Mahan G, Dabestani A, Gardin J, *et al*. Estimation of pulmonary artery pressure by pulsed Doppler echocardiography (abstract). *Circulation* 1983; 68(Suppl III):367.

Evaluation of the pericardium

Chirag R. Barbhaiya

Cardiovascular Diseases, Beth Israel Medical Center,
New York, NY, USA

CHAPTER 9

Echocardiography is the most important diagnostic modality in the management of pericardial diseases. It is extremely important to evaluate the pericardium during echocardiography, since it is a common cause of acute hemodynamic impairment.

The pericardium consists of an outer sac called the fibrous pericardium and a two-layered inner sac that creates a potential space surrounding the heart called the serous pericardium. A pericardial effusion appears on echocardiogram as an echo-free space between the two layers of serous pericardium.

Pericardial effusions

1 Result from an accumulation of fluid in the pericardial space [1].
2 Accumulation of >25 ml of fluid results in an effusion that is visible throughout the cardiac cycle.
3 "Trivial" effusions will be seen as a posterior echo-free space visible only in systole.
4 A pericardial effusion should be measured during diastole and is considered:
   • small: when its diameter is <1 cm,
   • medium: when its diameter is 1–2 cm
   • large: when its diameter is >2 cm.

Potential causes of pericardial effusions are listed in Table 9.1 in order of frequency of requiring pericardicentesis.

Practical Manual of Echocardiography in the Urgent Setting, First Edition.
Edited by Vladimir Fridman and Mario J. Garcia.
© 2013 John Wiley & Sons, Ltd. Published 2013 by John Wiley & Sons, Ltd.

Table 9.1 Causes of pericardial effusions requiring pericardiocentesis (all values %).

Malignant	34
Post-operative	25
Catheter-based procedure	10
Idiopathic	9
Other	5
Connective tissue disease	5
Infectious	4
Post-radiation	3
Ischemic	3
Renal failure	2

Echo-free spaces around the heart

Pericardial effusions are echo-free spaces that are usually located circumferentially and are larger posteriorly. There are, however, a number of other echo-free structures that must be differentiated from pericardial effusions.

- Pleural effusion – A posterior echo-free space that is posterior to the descending aorta is a pleural effusion. A pericardial effusion appears anterior to the descending aorta (Figure 9.1).
- Epicardial fat pad (Figure 9.2) – An echo-free space that is found only anteriorly. An anterior echo-free space without a posterior echo-free space is most likely an epicardial fat pad.
- Pericardial cyst (Figure 9.3) – An uncommon, benign structural abnormality of the pericardium that appears as a focal echo-free space most frequently in the right costo-phrenic angle. A pericardial cyst must be differentiated from a loculated pericardial effusion.

Cardiac tamponade

Cardiac tamponade represents one of the most important diagnoses to establish in the acute setting.

- Cardiac tamponade is a hemodynamic condition caused by accumulation of a pericardial effusion resulting in increased intrapericardial pressure that compromises filling of cardiac chambers and cardiac output.

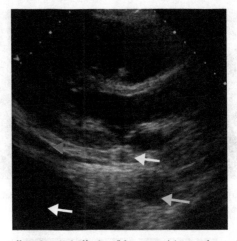

Figure 9.1 A small pericardial effusion (blue arrow) is noted anterior to the descending aorta (green arrow). A large pleural effusion (white arrow) is noted posterior to descending aorta. It is important to differentiate between the descending aorta (green arrow) and coronary sinus (yellow arrow) when determining between location of effusion.

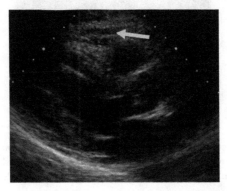

Figure 9.2 A small epicardial fat pad (arrow) is noted in this parasternal long axis view.

- Tamponade can be caused by a small amount of rapidly accumulating fluid.
- Various M-mode, 2D, and Doppler echocardiographic signs have been described to aid in the diagnosis of this life-threatening condition.

The first question to answer in a tamponade case is whether a pericardial effusion is present. Usually, the parasternal long axis view is a good starting point to answer this question (Figure 9.4).

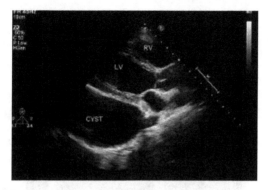

Figure 9.3 A large pericardiac cyst is noted (Reproduced from Thanneer *et al.* [2], with permission from Elsevier).

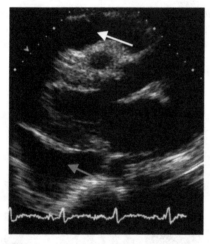

Figure 9.4 Parasternal long axis view showing a large pericardial effusion noted anterior to (white arrow) and posterior to (blue arrow) the heart. Note that the posterior portion of the pericardial effusion is not located posterior to the descending aorta.

Once the presence of a pericardial effusion has been established (irrespective of size), and if tamponade is clinically considered, multiple echocardiographic features of tamponade should be checked for:

1 Late diastolic RA collapse (Figure 9.5)
   - occurs when intrapericardial pressure exceeds the relatively low RA filling pressure;
   - the longer the duration of right atrial invagination relative to the length of the cardiac cycle, the greater the likelihood of significant hemodynamic compromise;

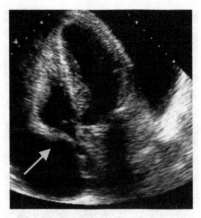

Figure 9.5 Diastolic collapse of the right atrium (arrow) is clearly present in this apical four-chamber view.

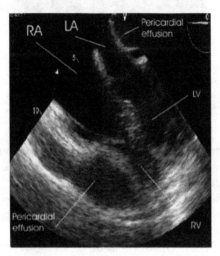

Figure 9.6 A TEE mid-esophageal four-chamber view showing collapse of the right ventricle in cardiac tamponade (Reproduced from Carmona *et al.* [6], with permission from Elsevier).

- inversion of the free wall of the right atrium for more than one-third of systole has a 94% sensitivity and 100% specificity for the diagnosis of tamponade [3];
- diastolic RA collapse may not occur if right heart pressures are elevated.
2 Early diastolic RV collapse (Figure 9.6)
   - occurs when intrapericardial pressure exceeds RV filling pressure, which is usually greater than RA filling pressure [4];

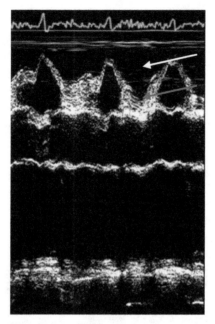

Figure 9.7 M-mode image of the LV. A pericardial effusion is noted anterior to the RVOT (white arrow), and a diastolic collapse of the RVOT is clearly noted (blue arrow).

- right ventricular diastolic collapse is a more specific, but less sensitive, indicator of hemodynamically significant pericardial compression [5];
- may not occur if right heart pressures are elevated;
- M-mode through the mid-ventricle can be performed from the parasternal long or short axis views and aids detection by improving temporal resolution;
  Figure 9.7 is an M-mode image which shows the presence of a pericardial effusion and a diastolic collapse of the right ventricle/RVOT;
- abnormal ventricular septal motion – septal shift and shudder;
- respiratory variation in ventricle chamber size – related to respiratory variation on ventricular filling; inspiratory increase in RV size with corresponding decrease in LV size most easily appreciated on M-mode;
- plethora of the IVC with blunted respiratory changes – increased right heart filling pressures caused by tamponade results in an IVC dilated >2cm with <50% change in diameter with respiration.

3 Respiratory variation in mitral inflow
- mitral inflow decreases during inspiration due to ventricular interdependence [7];

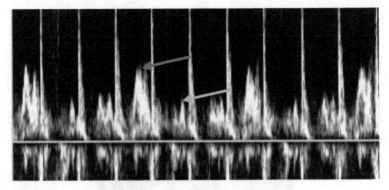

Figure 9.8 A PW Doppler scan of mitral inflow shows clearly that the difference in the peaks of E wave between the highest value (blue arrow) and lowest value (green arrow) varies by more than 25%, hinting toward the diagnosis of tamponade.

- PW of the mitral valve inflow is obtained at the level of the mitral valve leaflets and the sweep speed is lowered so multiple recordings of the inflow can be taken and respiratory variation can be recorded;
- a decrease in mitral inflow E velocity of >25% with inspiration is suggestive of cardiac tamponade (Figure 9.8); during positive pressure ventilation changes with inspiration are reversed;
- measurements should be made during one respiratory cycle.
- irregular rhythms such as atrial fibrillation or rhythms with frequent ventricular or atrial ectopy preclude reliable measurement of inflow velocity change.
4 Respiratory variation in tricuspid inflow
  - an increase in tricuspid inflow velocity of >50% during inspiration suggests cardiac tamponade (Figure 9.9) [7];
  - similar methods and considerations apply to measurement of tricuspid inflow as mitral inflow.
5 Pulmonary and hepatic venous flow velocity:
  - inspiratory decrease in pulmonary vein diastolic forward flow and inspiratory increase in hepatic forward flow suggest tamponade physiology.
  - isovolumic relaxation time (IVRT) lengthens with inspiration due to delayed opening of the mitral valve.

Echo-guided pericardiocentesis

The most effective treatment for cardiac tamponade is removal of pericardial fluid. Echochardiography can be used to guide pericardiocentesis by

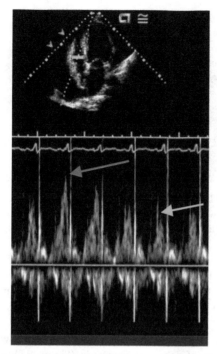

Figure 9.9 PW of the tricuspid valve inflow at the tricuspid valve leaflet level. The peak velocities of the second (blue arrow) and fifth (green arrow) beats were noted to be 50% different, hinting towards the diagnosis of tamponade.

locating the optimal site for puncture and determining distance from puncture site to pericardial effusion.

There are two approaches:

1 Subcostal window – the most commonly used
2 Apical window
   • Echocardiographic images are taken from the desired view.
   • Size and location of the pericardial effusion, and its relation to the location of the heart, are noted.
   • Real-time echocardiography can show the location of the catheter and its relation to the pericardial space and intracardiac structures (Figure 9.10).
• Agitated saline contrast can be used to show the location of the distal tip of the pericardiocentesis catheter (Figure 9.11).
• An extremely important part of pericardiocentesis is equipment set-up prior to the procedure. It is necessary to make sure that all the necessary equipment is available, and is properly set up, prior to performing the periocardiocentesis.

(a)

(b)

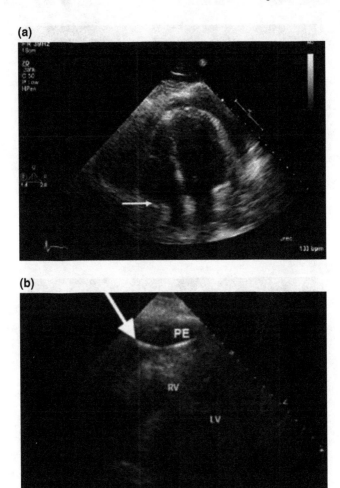

Figure 9.10 (a) Apical view showing a large pericardial effusion and RA collapse, indicative of tamponade; **(b)** echocardiography-guided pericardiocentesis was performed, with the catheter (arrow) noted in the pericardial space (Reproduced from Wann and Passen [8], with permission from Elsevier).

Constrictive pericarditis

Constrictive pericarditis may be a difficult, but important, diagnosis to make. It should be considered in patients with predominant right heart failure and a normal LV ejection fraction. Constrictive pericarditis is caused by a noncompliant pericardium. Common causes of constrictive pericarditis are listed it Table 9.2 in order of frequency.

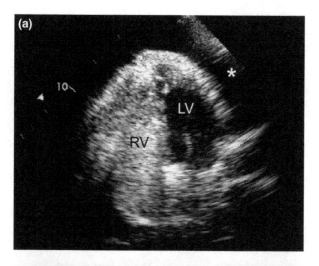

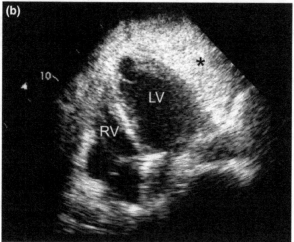

Figure 9.11 (a) During injection of agitated saline, opacification of right-sided chambers was noted, indicating that the distal tip of the catheter is inside one of these chambers; **(b)** pulling back of the catheter, and reinjection of agitated saline, showed opacification of pericardial space (asterisk), indicating the proper placement of the distal tip of the catheter within the pericardial space (Reproduced from Schussler and Grayburn [9], with permission from Elsevier).

The echocardiographic diagnosis is based on the detection of anatomical and physiological findings:

- Thickened pericardium – a thick pericardium is commonly seen. However, 20% of patients will have normal pericardial thickness.

Table 9.2 Causes of constrictive pericarditis (all values %).

Cardiac surgery	29
Idiopathic	26
Post-pericarditis	16
Radiation	11
Others	9
Collagen vascular	6
Infectious	3

- Rapid descend and flattening of the LV posterior wall during diastole – this finding is often best appreciated on M-mode.
- Abnormal ventricular septal motion and respiratory variation in ventricular size.
- Plethora of the IVC.
- Findings of respiratory variability and ventricular interdependence.

Although the underlying pathophysiology of constrictive pericarditis differs from that of cardiac tamponade, the resulting respiratory variation in hemodynamics and ventricular interdependence is similar. Thus, Doppler findings described in cardiac tamponade also suggest constrictive pericarditis, although with lower sensitivity and specificity.

Differentiation of constrictive pericarditis and restrictive cardiomyopathy [10]

Restrictive cardiomyopathies are primary myocardial disorders characterized by a restrictive filling pattern and reduced diastolic volume of the left or both ventricles with preserved ejection fraction. Although pathologically extremely different from constrictive pericarditis, patients with both types of disorders have very similar clinical presentations. It is extremely important to make the correct diagnosis in these patients, since the therapeutic approaches to these disorders are very different.

One of the most common restrictive cardiomyopathies is amyloidosis. The classic M-mode, parasternal long axis, and apical four-chamber views of a patient with amyloidosis are shown in Figure 9.12. When an echocardiogram has such an appearance, the diagnosis of amyloidosis must be considered in the differential diagnosis.

Specific hemodynamic parameters have been developed to aid in the differentiation of restrictive cardiomyopathy from constrictive pericarditis (Table 9.3).

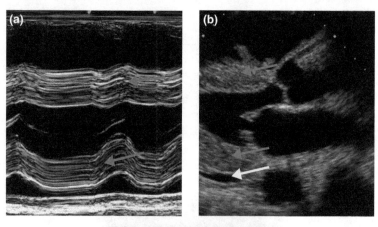

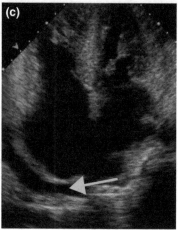

Figure 9.12 Echocardiographic features of amyloidosis: **(a)** M-mode view shows a typical "onion skin" appearance of the LV walls (blue arrows); **(b)** parasternal long axis view shows bright speckled LV walls (red arrows) and a presence of a small perciardial effusion (yellow arrow); **(c)** apical four-chamber view shows biatrial enlargement, normal ventricular size/systolic function, and a small pericardial effusion (green arrow).

Table 9.3 Hemodynamic features of constrictive pericarditis and restrictive cardiomyopathy.

	Constriction	Restriction
LVEDP-RVEDP (mm Hg)	≤5	>5
RV systolic pressure (mm Hg)	≤50	>50
RVEDP/RVSP (mm Hg)	≥0.33	<0.3

However, by echocardiography the differential diagnosis is based on the identification ventricular interdependence and preserved LV relaxation in constriction. When mitral inflow velocities suggest restrictive filling with E/A ratio >1.5 and/or a deceleration time <160 milliseconds, then a mitral septal annulus velocity >7 cm/s suggests constrictive pericarditis and is very rarely seen in restrictive cardiomyopathy.

A hepatic vein flow can also help in the differentiation of constriction versus. restriction:

- The sample volume of PW Doppler should be placed in the hepatic vein and the Doppler reading should be recorded at the same time as the patient's breathing pattern (inspiration and expiration) is noted and/or recorded.
  - ○ in both restriction and constriction, the forward flow in the hepatic vein is higher in diastole than in systole.
  - ○ diastolic flow reversal in restrictive cardiomyopathy is larger in inspiration whereas in constrictive pericarditis it is larger in expiration.

Effusive–constrictive pericarditis

Effusive–constrictive pericarditis results from a combination of pericardial effusion and constrictive pericarditis. To make the diagnosis of effusive–constrictive pericarditis, constrictive hemodynamics must persist after removal of pericardial fluid.

Overall, echocardiography is an extremely important tool toward diagnosing pericardial diseases, and is the initial test of choice in cases of possible cardiac tamponade. Although not specific to establish the cause of pericardial disease, echocardiography can aid in establishing the presence and severity of hemodynamic impairment and can guide further diagnostic and therapeutic interventions.

References

1 Soler-Soler J, Sagrista-Sauleda J, Permanyer-Miralda P. Management of pericardial effusion. *Heart* 2001; 86:235–40.
2 Thanneer L, Saric M, Perk G, *et al*. A giant pericardial cyst. *J Am Coll Cardiol* 2011; 57(17):1784.
3 Gillam LD, Guyer DE, Gibson TC, *et al*. Hydrodynamic compression of the right atrium: a new echocardiographic sign of tamponade. *Circulation* 1983; 68:294–301.
4 Singh S, Wann LS, Schuchard GH, *et al*. Right ventricular and right atrial collapse in patients with cardiac tamponade – a combined echocardiographic and hemodynamic study. *Circulation* 1984; 70:966–71.
5 Leimgruber PP, Klopfenstein HS, Wann LS, Brooks HL. The hemodynamic derangement associated with right ventricular diastolic collapse in cardiac tamponade: an experimental echocardiographic study. *Circulation* 1983; 68:612–20.

6 Carmona P, Mateo E, Casanovas I, *et al.* Management of cardiac tamponade after cardiac surgery. *J Cardiothorac Vasc Anesth* 2012; 26(2):302–11.

7 Gonzalez MS, Basnight MA, Appleton CP. Experimental pericardial effusion: relation of abnormal respiratory variation in mitral flow velocity to hemodynamics and diastolic right heart collapse. *J Am Coll Cardiol* 1991; 17(1):239–48.

8 Wann S, Passen E. Echocardiography is pericardial disease. *J Am Soc Echocardiogr* 2008; 2(1):7–13.

9 Schussler JM, Grayburn PA. Contrast guided two-dimensional echocardiography for needle localization during pericardiocentesis: a case report. *J Am Soc Echocardiogr* 2010; 23(6):683.e1–2.

10 Asher CR, Klein AL. Diastolic heart failure: restrictive cardiomyopathy, constrictive pericarditis, and cardiac tamponade: clinical and echocardiographic evaluation. *Cardiol Rev* 2002; 10(4):218–29.

Specialty echocardiographic examinations

Cesare Saponieri

Electrophysiology and Cardiovascular Diseases, New York, NY, USA

CHAPTER 10

In this chapter the application of echocardiography in unique clinical scenarios in the hospital setting is described.

TTE in a VAD patient

Ventricular assist devices (VADs) are mechanical circulatory devices that are placed by cardiac surgeons in cases of severe, treatment refractory, heart failure. They are designed to either assist the right ventricle (RVAD), left ventricle (LVAD), or both ventricles (BiVAD) of the heart. When initially introduced, these were very bulky devices but, over the recent years, have been gradually getting smaller. The locations of VADs have also drastically changed over the years. Initially, large bulky devices were placed in the abdominal cavity. However, most recent devices, which are about the size of a defibrillator, are placed within the thoracic cavity.

A graphical representation of one type of LVAD, and its placement in the human body, is shown in Figure 10.1.

The presence of a VAD poses many challenges to the echocardiographer:

- Identifying the type of VAD is difficult, especially if the proper history is not known, but is absolutely essential.
- As some VADs have a pulseless circulatory system, all standard volume/ flow equations, and Doppler measurements, become inaccurate.
- The acoustic windows are sometimes very limited with a lot of acoustic shadowing from the large metal devices.
- Cardiac output determinations are of limited use. The native LV stroke volume can be calculated from the LVOT pulsed Doppler, but the

Practical Manual of Echocardiography in the Urgent Setting, First Edition.
Edited by Vladimir Fridman and Mario J. Garcia.
© 2013 John Wiley & Sons, Ltd. Published 2013 by John Wiley & Sons, Ltd.

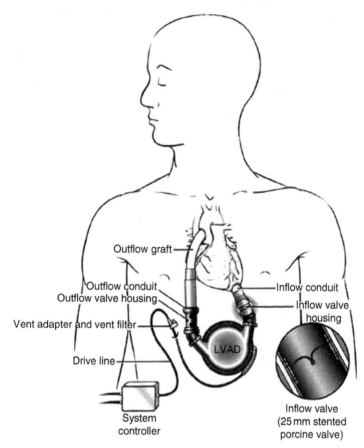

Figure 10.1 The placement of one type of LVAD device (Reproduced from Horton *et al.* [1], with permission from Elsevier).

augmented cardiac output provided by the VAD through the outflow cannula is difficult to quantify by Doppler.

- Normal LVAD function should be established with flow analysis (whether pulsatile or pulseless) at the insertion point of the LVAD outflow.
- In certain cases, the aortic valve may not open with every beat, or not open at all. This occurs when the LVAD is circulating the blood, and the native left ventricle is not capable of generating enough blood flow to open the valve.

In normal LVAD function:

- There is flow in the inflow (Figure 10.2) and outflow of the device.
- LV dimensions should not be significantly larger than pre-LVAD dimensions or too small to the point of cavity collapse.

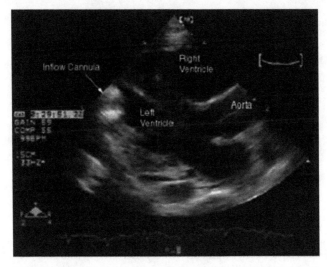

Figure 10.2 Parasternal long axis view of a heart with an LVAD device. The echocardiographic appearance of a properly positioned inflow cannula is noted in this figure (Reproduced from Horton *et al.* [1], with permission from Elsevier).

- Flow should be unidirectional.
- Specific Doppler characteristics of normal LVAD function can be found in the literature if needed [1].

Possible causes of LVAD malfunction or hemodynamic compromise in LVAD patients are:

- Inflow valve regurgitation.
- Inflow conduit obstruction.
- Outflow graft distortion/obstruction/regurgitation.
- Thrombosis within the device.
- Acquired native aortic valve disease [2].
- RV failure.
- Right-to-left shunting through a large patent foramen ovale (PFO).

Transesophageal echocardiogram (TEE) should be considered to more clearly evaluate LVAD function if clinically warranted. Transthoracic echocardiogram (TTE) examinations of any assist devices are extremely challenging, and should be performed by an experienced echocardiographer.

Intracardiac echocardiography

- In intracardiac echocardiography (ICE), a small mechanical rotational or phased array transducer inserted through a jugular or a femoral

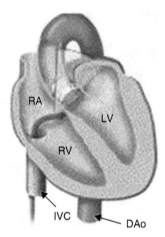

Figure 10.3 In this case, ICE is properly positioned to image a new percutaneous aortic valve replacement (Reproduced from Bartel *et al.* [4], with permission from Elsevier). DAo = descending aorta.

vein emits/receives ultrasound inside the heart. ICE is able to provide M-mode, 2D, and Doppler images [3].
- Catheters are tunneled through the venous system into the heart.
- The ICE catheter is placed inside the right chambers of the heart (Figure 10.3). From that position, views of almost all cardiac structures on right and left sides of the heart, such as crista terminalis, fossa ovalis and tricuspid valve apparatus, coronary artery stenoses, and venous and arterial inflows/outflows to the heart, can be obtained by rotation and flexion of the device.

Especially important is the use of ICE in the electrophysiology laboratory to guide complex electrophysiological procedures. The ICE device helps in positioning of ablation catheters. In ablations involving the left-sided cardiac structures, ICE can:
- Monitor trans-septal puncture.
- Help in visualizing the pulmonary veins.
- Guide proper ablation points.
- Monitor for serious complications.

Overall, the ICE system is extremely useful for real-time visualization of the heart (Figure 10.4). As opposed to using a TEE for the above stated purposes, the ICE system does not require prolonged intubation of the patient with a TEE probe, and does not require moderate/general sedation. However, it is limited by its invasive nature and the cost involved in this procedure.

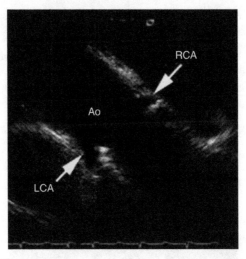

Figure 10.4 ICE is used to image clearly the takeoff of two coronary arteries above a newly placed percutaneous aortic valve (Reproduced from Bartel *et al.* [4], with permission from Elsevier). RCA = right coronary artery, LCA = left main coronary artery, Ao = aorta.

TEE in the operating room

Transesophageal echocardiogram, performed in the operating room (OR) by the case anesthesiologist or a cardiologist serves as the imaging modality of choice during a cardiothoracic surgery case.

- A standard transesophageal probe is passed down the esophagus, and a standard TEE is performed.
- The focus of the examination is usually to evaluate the structures of interest to the case. For example, during MV regurgitation surgery, all portions of the valve apparatus are carefully examined and serve as a guide to surgeons on how to proceed with the valve repair or replacement.

The TEE, as a procedure, is the same as a routine TEE discussed previously. The same equipment, technique, and views are utilized.

In most cases, an intraoperative TEE is used to determine the success of repair of cardiac structures on other structures within the heart. For example, in cases of simultaneous MV stenosis and tricuspid regurgitation, an intraoperative TEE is performed after the mitral valve is fixed to evaluate residual tricuspid valve regurgitation, and to further evaluate the tricuspid valve apparatus. The results of the TEE then guide the surgeons on whether to proceed with tricuspid valve surgery, or to conclude the procedure.

Echocardiography to guide percutaneous closure devices placement

These mesh-like devices are specifically manufactured to seal openings within the heart. These defects include:

- Atrial septal defects (Figures 10.5 and 10.6).
- Patent foramen ovale.

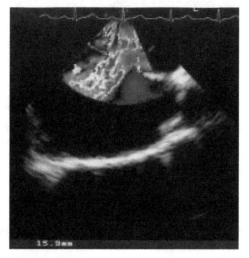

Figure 10.5 A TEE bicaval showing the presence of a secundum ASD defect (Reproduced from Thanapoulos *et al.* [5], with permission from Elsevier).

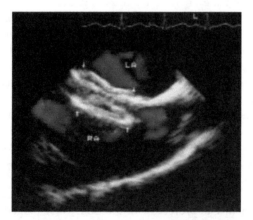

Figure 10.6 The appearance of the ASD from Figure 10.5 after a closure device has been applied (Reproduced from Thanapoulos *et al.* [5], with permission from Elsevier).

- Ventricular septal defects.
- Perivalvular leaks are capable of being closed percutaneously with closure devices. The exact role of percutaneous closure devices versus open heart surgery for the closure of such cardiac defects is still debated.

When percutaneous closure devices are used, their delivery and placement is tremendously aided by the use of transesophageal and/or intracardiac echocardiography [6].

References

1 Horton CS, Khodaverdian R, Chatelain P, *et al.* Left ventricular assist device malfunction: an approach to diagnosis by echocardiography. *J Am Coll Cardiol* 2005; 45:1435–40.
2 Rose AG, Park SJ, Bank AJ, *et al.* Partial aortic valve fusion induced by left ventricular assist device. *Ann Thorac Surg* 2000; 70:1270–4.
3 Packer DL, Stevens CL, Curley MG, *et al.* Intracardiac phased-array imaging: methods and initial clinical experience with high resolution, under blood visualization: initial experience with intracardiac phased-array ultrasound. *J Am Coll Cardiol* 2002; 39:509–16.
4 Bartel T, Bonaros N, Muller L, *et al.* Intracardiac echocardiography: a new guiding tool for transcatheter aortic valve replacement. *J Am Soc Echocar* 2011; 24(9):966–75.
5 Thanapoulos BD, Laskari CV, Tsaousis GS, *et al.* Closure of atrial septal defects with the amplatzer occlusion device: preliminary results. *J Am Coll Cardiol* 1998; 31(5):1110–6.
6 Hijazi ZM, Wang Z, Qi-Ling C, *et al.* Transcatheter closure of atrial septal defects and patent foramen ovale under intracardiac echocardiographic guidance: Feasibility and comparison with transesophageal echocardiography. *Cathet Cardiovasc Intervent* 2001; 52(2):194–9.
   Thanapoulos BD, Laskari CV, Tsaousis GS, *et al.* Closure of Atrial Septal Defects With the Amplatzer Occlusion Device: Preliminary Results. *J Amer Coll Cardiol* 1998;31(5):1110–6.

Common artifacts

Padmakshi Singh[1], Moinakhtar Lala[2], and Sapan Talati[3]

[1]Cardiovascular Diseases, SUNY Downstate Medical Center, New York, NY, USA
[2]Cardiovascular Diseases, Beth Israel Medical Center, New York, NY, USA
[3]SUNY Downstate Medical Center, Brooklyn, New York, NY, USA

CHAPTER 11

When performing an echocardiogram, it is extremely important to distinguish between actual anatomical structures and artifacts. Artifacts are displayed images that do not accurately represent true anatomical structures or hemodynamics.

It is vital for the echocardiographer to recognize artifacts, as they can appear as very serious pathological conditions, and can lead to the incorrect diagnosis and treatment of patients [1].

There are three types of artifacts [2]:

1 Artifacts that alter the size and/or shape of structures.
2 Artifacts that create the appearance of structures that are not physically present.
3 Artifacts that hide the appearance of structures that are physically present.

Artifacts are generated by the combination of physical properties of the ultrasound beam and their interaction with the body and algorithms that convert the ultrasound information received by the transducer into images. These algorithms usually assume that the ultrasound wave that left the transducer traveled a straight path to the object being imaged, and then returned on a straight path to the transducer at a constant speed. Obviously, that is not the case for many ultrasound waves that enter the human body and, therefore, artifacts are a frequent occurrence in echocardiography and general medical ultrasound imaging.

The most common echocardiographic artifacts are explained here.

- Propagation speed artifacts – the ultrasound machine assumes that all signals travel at a speed of 1540 m/s in the body, the speed of sound

Practical Manual of Echocardiography in the Urgent Setting, First Edition.
Edited by Vladimir Fridman and Mario J. Garcia.
© 2013 John Wiley & Sons, Ltd. Published 2013 by John Wiley & Sons, Ltd.

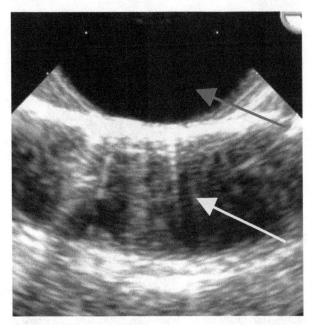

Figure 11.1 Mirror image artifact of the descending aorta. The second lumen (yellow arrow) is an artifact arising from the true aortic lumen (blue arrow).

propagation in water. When the ultrasound goes through objects that have a different propagating velocity, such as air or bone, the structures distant to the object are placed incorrectly in space.

- Mirror image (Figure 11.1) – strong reflectors result in the structures that are in proximity to the transducer reappearing again at a multiple of the actual depth. This occurs because part of the strong signal is reflected again at the transducer crystal surface when received. A common appearance of this artifact is when the aorta is being imaged during a TEE, there appears to be two aortas on the screen – one at the back of the other [3].
- Reverberation (Figure 11.2) – the appearance of lines of increasing depth at even intervals, due to the presence of two strong reflectors, with the ultrasound wave bouncing back and forth between these reflectors, prior to coming back to the receiving transducer.
- Comet tail (Figure 11.3) – a form of reverberation that occurs when there is a large difference in acoustic impedance between a very strong reflecting object and its surroundings. The artifact appears as two tails arising from a structure, resembling a comet.
- Refraction (Figure 11.4) – distortions of images due to the bending of ultrasound beams as they pass from one medium to another.

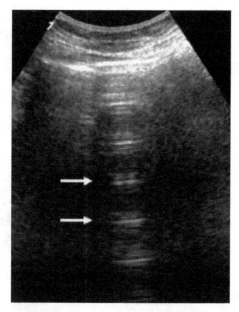

Figure 11.2 Reverberation artifact (arrows) are noted distal to a strong proximal reflector (Reproduced from Sperandeo *et al.* [4]).

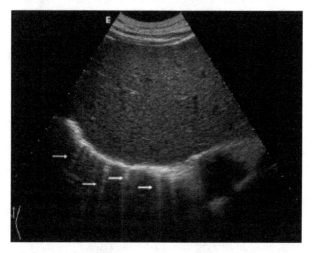

Figure 11.3 Comet tail artifacts (arrows) are noted along the border of structures with different acoustic properties (Reproduced from Sperandeo *et al.* [4]).

An important example of this is Ghost image artifact: the presence of refraction creates almost two separate, but side-by-side, images of the same structure. This is different from mirror artifact, where the two images are placed one on top of the other.

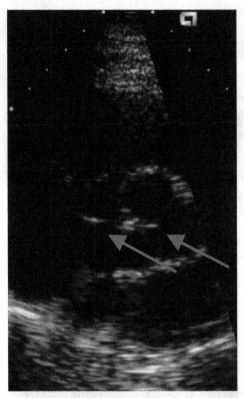

Figure 11.4 A refraction artifact causes the appearance of two side by side aortic valves (arrows) in this parasternal short axis view (Reproduced from Spieker *et al.* [5], with permission from Elsevier).

- Side lobes (Figure 11.5) – arise due to the presence of pulses that travel out of the transducer in a direction that is not parallel to the main pulse. These pulses then come back to the transducer, which assumes that the ultrasound traveled in the same direction as the main pulse, and misplaces the location of the structures that reflected these aberrant pulses.
- Shadowing (Figure 11.6) – the presence of highly reflective structures, such as calcium or mechanical valves, prevents the ultrasound from traveling to structures behind these strong reflectors, and thus hides all of these distal structures.
- Acoustic enhancement (Figure 11.7) – fluid-filled structures attenuate the ultrasound wave less than solid structures. As such, structures distal to fluid receive, and thus reflect, more ultrasound energy than the same structures, at the same distances, with only solid tissues proximal to them. The ultrasound probe then receives much higher

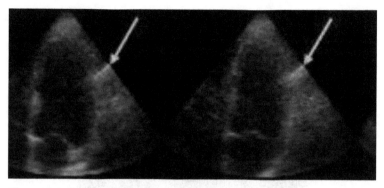

Figure 11.5 Side lobes artifacts are seen in these apical views (Reproduced from Leung *et al.* [6], with permission from Elsevier).

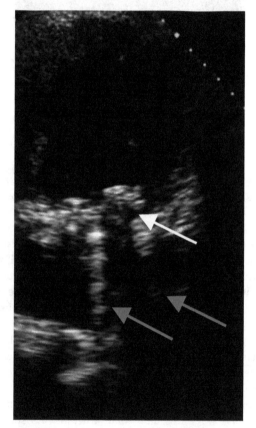

Figure 11.6 Shadowing (blue arrows) from a mechanical mitral valve (white arrow) is seen in this figure. Due to the shadowing profile of this valve, it can be concluded that it is a St Jude's mechanical prosthetic valve.

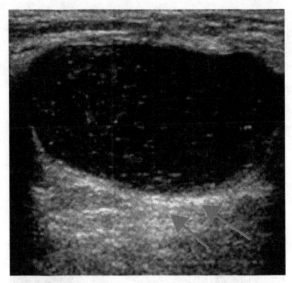

Figure 11.7 Bright echos (arrows) are seen distal to a fluid-filled structure due to the presence of acoustic enhancement (Reproduced from Cardenosa [7], with permission from Elsevier).

energy signals from structures behind fluid than from those behind solids, and shows the structures behind fluid as much more echogenic than they really are.

Use of color and spectral Doppler has also introduced new type of artifacts to the field of echocardiography. It is extremely important for the observer to be aware of such artifacts to correctly interpret flows and fluid movements in the presence of these artifacts.

- Overgain/undergain – these are described in detail in Chapter 1. In general, different Doppler gain settings can result in drastically different Doppler images. Flows can be hidden with undergaining and flows that do not exist can appear with overgaining. When choosing the gain settings, the general rule is: gain should be set just slightly below the level when signal appears inside the background tissues.
- Twinkling artifact – is seen as a line containing rapidly changing red and blue colors behind a strongly reflective structure (Figure 11.8) [8]. In echocardiography, this usually arises behind calcified valves, and can lead to false readings of valvular regurgitation.
- Aliasing – appearance of multiple colors in high velocity flows (described further in Chapter 1) (Figures 11.9 and 11.10).

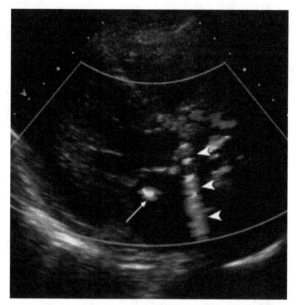

Figure 11.8 A twinkling artifact is noted behind a calcified aortic valve (arrowheads). Mild mitral regurgitation (arrow) is noted, and should not be confused with the twinkling artifact (Reproduced from Tsao *et al.* [9], with permission from Elsevier).

- Flow reversal – the thin area between two flows going in opposite directions is visualized as a black line, which artifactually indicates that no flow occurs in the region (Figure 11.10).
- Doppler angle – accurate estimations of velocities can be performed by Doppler only if the Doppler angle is correctly measured/estimated. Slight variations in the Doppler angle can produce drastic differences in the velocities obtained on Doppler analysis (as described in detail in Chapter 1).

These, and other, artifacts can severely distort ultrasound images and obtained calculations, and in many cases, can pose diagnostic and treatment dilemmas. When it is unclear whether certain structures/flows are real or artifacts, multiple views of these structures and multiple measurements of these flows should be obtained. As a rule of thumb, artifacts disappear when imaged from other angles and views, while real structures are not altered. It is thus critical that echocardiographers are aware of, and can recognize, artifacts, so that misdiagnoses arising from artifacts are avoided and the correct conclusions are drawn from the echocardiogram images.

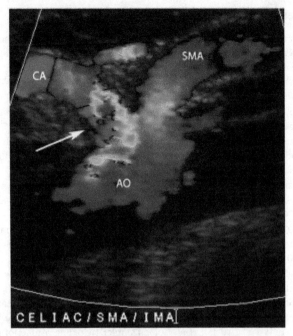

Figure 11.9 High grade stenosis, and resulting high velocities of blood through the stenotic artery, results in an aliasing artifact (arrow), as seen by multiple different color flows in the stenotic segment (Reproduced from Revzin and Pellerito [10], with permission from Elsevier).

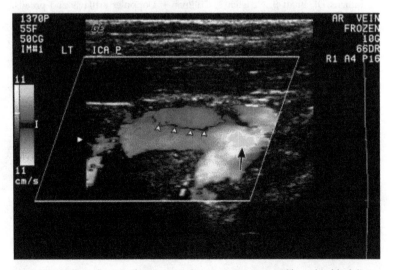

Figure 11.10 Two flows in the opposite directions are separated by a thin black line, which artifactually indicates no flow in that area (arrowheads). Aliasing artifact is also noted (arrow) (Reproduced from Rubens *et al.* [11], with permission from Elsevier).

References

1 DeMaria AN, Bommer W, Joye JA, Mason DT. Cross-sectional echocardiography: physical principles, anatomic planes, limitations and pitfalls. *Am J Cardiol* 1980; 46(7):1097–108.
2 Allen MN. *Echocardiography*, 2nd edn. Philadelphia: Lippincott, Williams & Wilkins, 1999.
3 Appelbe AF, *et al*. Clinical significance and origin of artifacts in transesophageal echocardiography of the thoracic aorta. *J Am Coll Cardiol* 1993; 21(3):754–60.
4 Sperandeo M, Varriale A, Sperandeo G, *et al*. Characterization of the normal pulmonary surface and pneumonectomy space by reflected ultrasound. *J Ultras* 2011; 14:22–7.
5 Spieker LE, Hufschmid U, Oechslin E, Jenni R. Double aortic and pulmonary valves: an artifact generated by ultrasound refraction. *J Am Soc Echo* 2004;17 (7)787–7.
6 Leung KYE, Danilouchkine MG, van Stralen M, *et al*. Probabilistic framework for tracking in artifact-prone 3D echocardiograms. *Med Im Analys* 2010; 14:750–8.
7 Cardenosa G. Cysts, cystic lesions, and papillary lesions. *Ultrasound Clinics* 2006; 1(4):617–29.
8 Rahmouni A, Bargoin R, Herment A, *et al*. Color Doppler twinkling artifact in hyperechoic regions. *Radiology* 1996; 199(1):269–71.
9 Tsao TF, Wu YL, Yu JM, *et al*. Color Doppler twinkling artifact of calcified cardiac valves in vitro: a not well known phenomenon in echocardiography. *Ultrasound Med Biol* 2011; 37(3):386–92.
10 Revzin MV, Pellerito JS. Ultrasound assessment of the mesenteric arteries. *Ultrasound Clinics* 2007; 2(3):477–92.
11 Rubens DJ, Bhatt S, Nedelka S, Cullinan J, Dopppler artifacts and pitfalls. *Ultrasound Clinics* 2006;1(1):79–109.

Hypotension and shock

Sheila Gupta Nadiminti

Department of Cardiology, Beth Israel Medical Center, New York, NY, USA

Transthoracic echocardiography (TTE) may be used to obtain significant hemodynamic information. Although physical exam and invasive monitoring can provide detailed information about critically ill patients, echocardiography has emerged as a safe, noninvasive and effective technique for diagnosis and monitoring of these patients.

Determination of central venous pressure, stroke volume, cardiac output, and vascular resistance

The determination of cardiac output, stroke volume and ventricular filling pressures are important clinically for the diagnosis and management of various hemodynamic conditions.

Stroke volume
- Stroke volume (SV) is a determinant of cardiac output (CO=HR×SV).
- It is used to calculate ejection fraction (EF=SV/LVEDV).
- The SV can be determined from 2D apical images:

$$SV = end-diastolic\ volume(EDV) - end-systolic\ volume(ESV)$$

  where EDV and ESV are determined using the biplane Simpson's method. If there is mitral regurgitation (MR), the regurgitant volume needs to be subtracted to obtain the effective SV [1]. The SV obtained by 2D is often underestimated if there is apical foreshortening.
- The LVOT stroke volume can be obtained using the LVOT area (Pi×radius squared) multiplied by the pulsed Doppler LVOT VTI. This

Practical Manual of Echocardiography in the Urgent Setting, First Edition.
Edited by Vladimir Fridman and Mario J. Garcia.

Doppler method is in most cases the most reproducible and reliable method in the acute care setting.

Filling pressures

The most reliable method to estimate LV filling pressures is the Doppler E/E' ratio (Figure 12.1) (as described in Chapter 4):

- E/E' >15 →LA pressure >15 mm Hg.
- E/E' <8 →LA pressure normal.
- If 8 < E/E' < 15, then other techniques such as pulmonary vein, flow duration and Valsalva can help to identify filling pressures [2].
- Make sure the same units are used for E and E' in the calculation of the E/E' ratio.

Pulmonary vascular resistance (PVR) and systemic vascular resistance (SVR)

PVR in echocardiography can be estimated by the formula (Figure 12.2):

$$\text{PVR estimation} = (\text{peak Tricuspid Regurgitation Jet Velocity}) / \text{RVOT TVI}$$

- A value above 0.175 has a 77% sensitivity and 81% specificity to identify PVR >2 Woods units [3].
- Normal PVR values are 20–130 dyn s/cm^5 or 0.25–1.6 Woods units.
- Standard conversion between absolute resistance units and Woods units is:

$$\text{Absolute resistance units} = \text{Woods units} \times 80$$

SVR in echocardiography can be estimated by the formula (Figure 12.3):

$$\text{SVR estimation} = (\text{peak Mitral Regurgitation Jet Velocity}) / \text{LVOT VTI}$$

- A value above 0.27 has a 70% sensitivity and 77% specificity to identify SVR >14 Woods units [4].
- A value below 0.2 has a 92% sensitivity and 88% specificity to identify SVR <10 Woods units [4].
- Normal SVR values are 700–1600 dyn s/cm^5 (absolute resistance units) or 9–20 Wood units.

Hypovolemia

Assessment of the IVC aids in measuring right atrial pressure (RAP). The IVC is a compliant vessel whose size varies with changes in intravascular pressure. The IVC collapses with inspiration as the blood is pumped out of the IVC due to the negative pressure created by chest expansion. In healthy subjects breathing spontaneously, cyclic changes in thoracic pressure result in collapse of the IVC diameter of

(a)

(b)

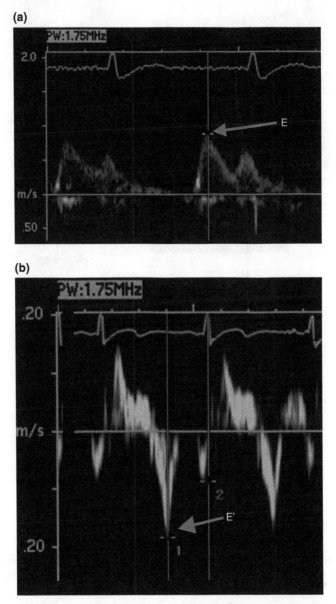

Figure 12.1 **(a)** E as derived from the PW Doppler of mitral inflow; **(b)** E′ as derived from the tissue Doppler of the lateral portion of the mitral valve annulus.

approximately 50% [5]. The subcostal view with the patient in the supine position is the best position for making measurements. The IVC is in long axis and measurements are made at end expiration (Figure 12.4).

(a)

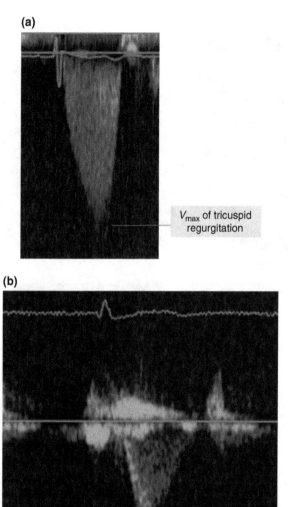

V_{max} of tricuspid
regurgitation

(b)

Figure 12.2 (a) The point corresponding to V_{max} of tricuspid regurgitation and
(b) the RVOT VTI are needed for calculation of PVR. RVOT VTI is obtained by
using PW Doppler in the parasternal short axis view of the base of the heart.

The diameter on inspiration and expiration are measured approximately
1 cm distal to the IVC–hepatic vein junction where the anterior and posterior walls are clearly visualized [6]. As RA pressure increases, this is
transmitted to the IVC, resulting in reduced collapse with inspiration
and IVC dilatation.

(a)

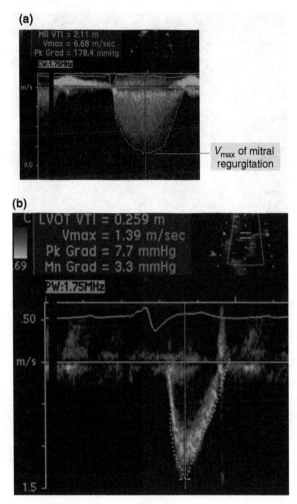

V_max of mitral regurgitation

(b)

Figure 12.3 (a) The point corresponding to V_{max} of mitral regurgitation and **(b)** tracing of the LVOT VTI are needed for calculation of SVR. The LVOT VTI is obtained by using PW Doppler in the apical five-chamber view at the LVOT.

Chapter 4 describes cutoffs for RAP based on IVC size. As the pressure in the right atrium increases, the pressure in the vena cava surpasses the respiratory pressure changes, so less dilation occurs. In scenarios in which IVC diameter and collapse do not fit this paradigm, an intermediate value of 8 mm Hg (range 5–10 mm Hg) may be used or secondary indices of elevated RA pressure should be integrated. These include:
- restrictive right-sided diastolic filling pattern;
- tricuspid E/E′ ratio >6;

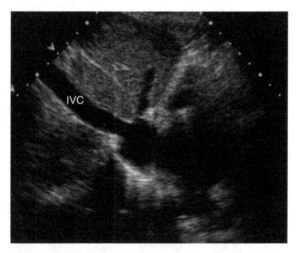

Figure 12.4 View of the IVC from the subcostal view (as seen in Chapter 2).

- diastolic flow predominance in the hepatic veins (which can be quantified as a systolic filling fraction <55%);
- if none of these secondary indices of elevated RA pressure are present, RA pressure may be downgraded to 3 mm Hg [7].

Exceptions to these rules are:
- in normal young athletes, the IVC may be dilated in the presence of normal pressure;
- in patients requiring ventilatory support, the IVC is commonly dilated and should not be used in such cases to estimate RA pressure;
- in complex cases, the SVR can be calculated as described above. In case of hypovolemia, the SVR is high, and a low SVR should steer the interpreting physician to a different diagnosis.

Septic shock

Septic shock is characterized by low or normal RA pressure, low SVR and low, normal or high stroke volume.
- RA pressure should be measured via the IVC.
- SVR and PVR should be calculated.
- Sepsis-induced myocardial dysfunction can be diagnosed, and responses to therapy can be monitored with echocardiography. Myocardial depression may be reversible [9, 10]. Depressed LV systolic function is associated with normal or low LV filling pressure, unlike the "classic" pattern of cardiogenic shock where LV pressures are elevated [11, 12].

- Patients with persistent shock should be evaluated for left and/or right heart failure, dynamic left ventricular obstruction, or tamponade if they do not respond to resuscitation and norepinephrine [8].

Cardiogenic shock due to left ventricular failure

There are multiple causes of cardiogenic shock. The most common causes are:
- myocardial infarction
- mechanical complication of myocardial infarction
- right ventricular infarction
- cardiomyopathy and myocarditis
- flow obstruction

Cardiogenic shock is defined as hypotension and prolonged tissue hypoperfusion due to cardiac dysfunction in the presence of adequate left ventricular filling pressure and volume. A cardiac index below 1.8l/min/m² is indicative of cardiogenic shock. The most common cause of cardiogenic shock is acute myocardial infarction. In the setting of a large myocardial infarction, pulmonary artery wedge pressure generally exceeds 25mm Hg and has an in-hospital mortality rate of at least 15–20% [13]. Cardiogenic shock is associated with a high SVR. Cardiogenic shock occurs when 40% or more of the left ventricle is infarcted. Cardiogenic shock usually occurs within hours of infarction due to ischemia and necrosis [14].

In cardiogenic shock, echocardiography provides information on:
- LV chamber size
- Overall systolic function and regional wall motion abnormalities.

Echocardiography is also useful to aid in other alternative diagnosis such as:
- cardiac tamponade
- hypertrophic obstructive cardiomyopathy
- acute or chronic valvular abnormalities.

Cardiogenic shock due to right ventricular failure

Cardiogenic shock due to right ventricular infarction alone is rare. RV infarction is difficult to diagnose on echocardiography, as the right ventricle is frequently not completely and clearly visualized. TAPSE, as described in Chapter 6, can be used as a quantitative measure of RV function, and a value of <1.8 cm is associated with RV systolic dysfunction.

Most RV infarctions involve part of the left ventricle as well. Therapy for RV infarction involves volume expansion with careful use of inotropes and differentiation from other forms of shock is crucial due to difference in the management. Hemodynamically, patients with RV infarction usually have normal or low RV systolic pressure, pulmonary artery diastolic pressures and pulmonary wedge pressure.

Cardiogenic shock due to acute valvular insufficiency or shunt

Acute severe mitral regurgitation causes a sudden overload of left atrial and left ventricular volumes. This leads to a decrease in stroke volume and lower cardiac output. Pulmonary vascular congestion and cardiogenic shock can develop. Causes of acute severe MR include:
- myocardial infarction
- endocarditis
- papillary muscle rupture or trauma.

Echocardiography can evaluate the structure of the mitral valve and look for clues as to the cause, including flail leaflets and a ruptured papillary muscle. Acute mitral regurgitation is associated with substantial elevation of left atrial pressure. This results in the classic "cut-off sign" on Doppler (Figure 12.5). This is indicative of rapid equalization of LA and LV pressures due to severe MR. With chronic MR, the left atrium dilates and compliance increases.

Acute aortic insufficiency (AI) is often caused by:
- endocarditis
- aortic dissection
- chest trauma

In acute AI, volume overload is poorly tolerated because the left ventricle has no time to remodel to accommodate the increase in volume. LV diastolic pressure rises rapidly, which may lead to premature closure of the mitral valve (seen on M-mode). There is a rapid rate of deceleration of the AI jet (Figure 12.6).

Acute pulmonary hypertension/ pulmonary embolism

Early detection and aggressive management are key in reducing death from PE. High-risk PE, presenting with hypotension, shock, RV dysfunction or right heart thrombus is associated with a high mortality, particularly during the first few hours. Despite modern methods for diagnosis and treatment, the mortality rate can be as high as 30% in patients presenting with massive PE [18]. Echocardiography is not indicated to establish the diagnosis but is used to risk stratify patients with PE. Poor prognostic indicators include:
- hypotension
- presence of patent foramen ovale (PFO)

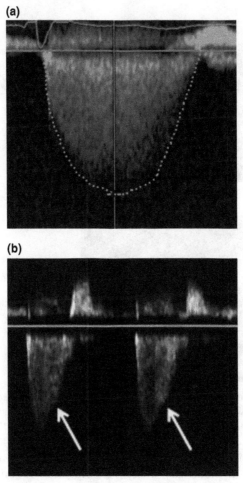

Figure 12.5 (a) CW Doppler of mild-to-moderate MR jet. **(b)** In severe acute MR, the jet has an abrupt cutoff (cut-off sign) (arrow) [15]. This CW Doppler pattern (arrows) is further elucidated in experimental models (Reproduced from Chetboul and Tissier [16], with permission from Elsevier).

- free floating right heart thrombus
- right heart dysfunction.

In patients with major PE (with associated RV dysfunction), detection of right-to-left shunt through a PFO signifies a higher risk of death and arterial thromboembolic complications. Patients with a PFO also had a significantly higher incidence of ischemic stroke and peripheral arterial embolism [19, 20]. In addition, serial imaging of right ventricular function can help physicians monitor the effect of treatment and judge whether the selected management strategy is successful.

(a)

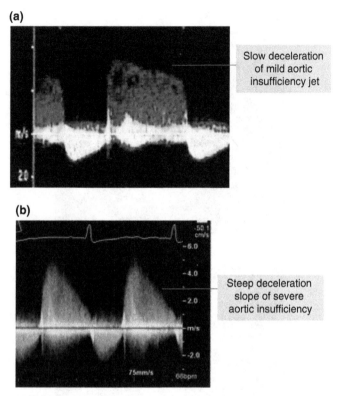

Slow deceleration of mild aortic insufficiency jet

(b)

Steep deceleration slope of severe aortic insufficiency

Figure 12.6 (a) In mild aortic insufficiency, the AI jet has a gradual deceleration slope [15]. However, in severe aortic insufficiency, (b) the AI jet is noted to have a steep deceleration slope (Reproduced from Kirkpatrick and Lang [17]).

With massive PE, the increase in right ventricular wall tension caused by the rise in pulmonary artery pressure leads to impaired right ventricular function and dilatation of the RV. A pulmonary embolus should be suspected if TTE reveals:

- right sided chamber dilatation;
- RV dysfunction;
- IVC which is dilated and unreactive;
- tricuspid regurgitation and/or elevated PA pressures – severe pulmonary hypertension is only present if there is previous chronic PE or other causes;
- small LV cavity, often hyperdynamic.

A distinct echocardiographic pattern of RV dysfunction, with akinesia of the RV free wall but normal motion at apex, has been shown to occur in acute PE and has been coined "McConnell's sign" (this is discussed further in Chapter 13) [21].

Another sign, known as the "60/60" sign, can help aid in the diagnosis of PE:

60/60 sign = Pulmonary ejection acceleration time in RVOT < 60 ms in the presence of tricuspid insufficiency pressure gradient < 60 mm Hg.

In summary, the important things to check for or determine in a hypotension/shock case are:
- LV ejection fraction
- cardiac output/stroke volume
- RV volumes and function
- SVR
- PVR
- presence of wall motion abnormalities
- any acute/severe valvular abnormalities
- estimate right atrial and pulmonary artery pressures
- if possible, determine the LVEDP and left atrial pressures
- rule out emergent cardiac conditions (such as pulmonary embolus, LV muscle rupture).

References

1 Oh JK, Seward JB, Tajik AJ. *The Echo Manual*. New York: Wolters Kluwer/ Lippincott, Williams & Wilkins, 2006.

2 Mather PJ. *Jefferson Heart Institute Handbook of Cardiology*. Sandbury, MA: Jones & Bartlett Learning, 2011.

3 Abbas AE, Fortuin FD, Schiller NB, *et al.* A simple method for noninvasive estimation of pulmonary vascular resistance. *J Am Col Cardiol* 2003; 41(6):1021–7.

4 Abbas AE, Fortuin FD, Patel B, *et al.* Noninvasive measurement of systemic vascular resistance using Doppler echocardiography. *J Am Soc Echocar* 2004; 17(8):834–8.

5 Pinsky MR, Brochard L, Macebo J. *Applied Physiology in Intensive Care Medicine*, 2nd edn. New York: Springer-Verlag, 2009.

6 Lyon M. *Beyond Fast*. Atlanta, GA: Medical College of Georgia, 2008.

7 Rudski LG, Lai WW, Afilalo J, *et al.* Guidelines for the echocardiographic assessment of the right heart in adults. *J Am Soc Echcoardiogr* 2010; 23:685–713.

8 Parker M, Shelhamer J, Bacharach S, *et al.* Profound but reversible myocardial depression in patients with septic shock. *Ann Intern Med* 1984; 100:483–90.

9 Parrillo JE, Burch C, Shelhamer JH, *et al.* A circulating myocardial depressant substance in humans with septic shock. septic shock patients with a reduced ejection fraction have a circulating factor that depresses *in vitro* myocardial cell performance. *J Clin Invest* 1985; 76:1539–53.

10 Jardin F, Brun-Ney D, Auyert B, *et al.* Sepsis-related cardiogenic shock. *Crit Care Med* 1990; 18:1055–60.

11 Bouhemad B, Nicolas-Robin A, Arbelot C, *et al*. Acute left ventricular dilatation and shock-induced myocardial dysfunction. *Crit Care Med* 2009; 37:441–47.

12 Griffee MJ, Merkel MJ, Wei KS. The role of echocadriography in hemodynamic assessment of septic shock. *Crit Care Clin* 2010; 26(2):365–82.

13 Fuster VR, Alexander W, O'Rourke RA. *Hurst's The Heart, Book 1*. New York: McGraw-Hill Companies, Inc., 2011.

14 Hochman JS. Cardiogenic shock complicating acute myocardial infarction – etiologies, management and outcome: A report from the SHOCK Trial Registry. *J Am Coll Cardiol* 2000; 36:1063–70.

15 Zoghbi WA, Enriquez-Sarano M, Foster E, *et al*. Recommendations for evaluation of the severity of native valvular regurgitation with two-dimensional and Doppler echocardiography. *J Am Soc Echocardiogr* 2003; 16(7):777–802.

16 Chetboul V, Tissier R. Echocardiographic assessment of canine degenerative mitral valve disease. *J Vet Cardiol* 2012; 14(1):127–48.

17 Kirkpatrick JN, Lang RM. Surgical echocardiography of heart valves: A primer for the cardiovascular surgeon. *Sem Thor Card Surg* 2010; 22(3):200.e1–22.

18 Fedullo P, Tapson V. The Evaluation of Suspected Pulmonary Embolism. *N Engl J Med* 2003; 349:1247–56.

19 Konstantinides S, Geibel A, Kasper W, *et al*. Patent foramen ovale is an important predictor of adverse outcomes in patients with major pulmonary embolism. *Circulation* 1998; 97(19):1946–51.

20 Torbiscki A, Perrier A, Konstantinides S, *et al*. Guidelines on the diagnosis and management of acute pulmonary embolism: The task force for the diagnosis and management of acute pulmonary embolism of the European Society of Cardiology. *Eur Heart J* 2008; 29:2276–315.

21 McConnell MV, Solomon SD, Rayan ME, *et al*. Regional right ventricular dysfunction detected by echocardiography in acute pulmonary embolism. *Am J Cardiol* 1996; 78:496–73.

Chest pain syndrome

Sandeep Dhillon and Jagdeep Singh

Cardiovascular Diseases, Beth Israel Medical Center, New York, NY, USA

Chest pain syndrome is one of the most common causes of emergency room visits and hospital admissions. Chest pain can be caused by multiple body systems and organs, and can range from benign costochondritis to life-threatening aortic dissection.

The three most important diagnoses to consider in any chest pain patient are:

1 Myocardial infarction
2 Aortic dissection
3 Pulmonary embolus.

Echocardiography is an essential diagnostic tool in the evaluation of acute chest pain cases, since there are features on a routine echocardiogram which can suggest, or rule out, any of the three diagnoses.

Myocardial Infarction

It is possible to diagnose an infarction on an echocardiogram. A critical finding is the presence of regional wall motion abnormalities, which are almost always linked to coronary artery disease/ischemia, and can even be related to a specific coronary artery distribution (Figure 13.1) [1, 2]. It is important to remember that the presence of wall motion abnormalities can be acute or chronic, and can also be caused by other myocardial processes. However, preserved wall thickness in an akinetic or hypokinetic segment suggests a recent event.

When performing an echocardiogram in an MI case, it is important to pay attention to all wall motion segments and all valves. Any hypokinesis/

Practical Manual of Echocardiography in the Urgent Setting, First Edition.
Edited by Vladimir Fridman and Mario J. Garcia.
© 2013 John Wiley & Sons, Ltd. Published 2013 by John Wiley & Sons, Ltd.

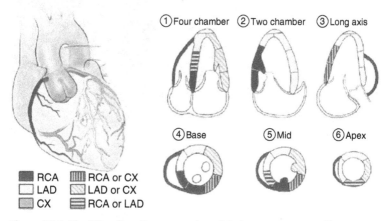

Figure 13.1 The LV wall motion segments and their coronary artery disease distribution (Reproduced from [2], with permission from Elsevier).

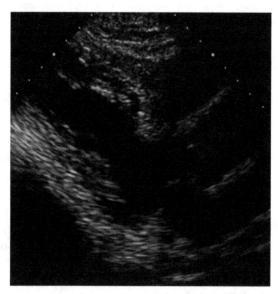

Figure 13.2 Parasternal long axis view in diastole in a case of anterior STEMI.

akinesis should be noted, as well as any possible acute valvular regurgitation.

As rules of thumb:

- If an LV wall segment is hypokinetic/akinetic, but is not thinned out (Figures 13.2 and 13.3), it is likely ischemic.

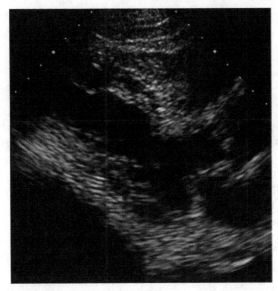

Figure 13.3 Systolic frame of the same case shown in Figure 13.2. Note the mid-anteroseptal wall is not contracting due to acute ischemia, but is not thinned out, indicating either a recent process or viable myocardium.

- If an LV wall segment is akinetic and is thinned out, it is likely to be nonviable tissue.

Golden Rule: in a ST-elevation MI case, never postpone angiography to perform an echocardiogram unless a specific need for an echo arises (such as to rule out tamponade etc.). If echo is performed, make sure:

- All wall segments are noted.
- Any wall motion abnormalities are recorded.
- All valves are interrogated.
- Draw conclusions only after ALL views are performed, as "quick" parasternal views can miss many wall motion abnormalities.

A grading system, the Wall Motion Score Index (WMSI), has been developed to indicate the severity of the wall motion abnormalities present on the echocardiogram [3].

The contractility of all of the 17 ASE LV wall motion segments are graded:

1 Normal motion
2 Hypokinetic segment
3 Akinetic segment
4 Dyskinetic segment

WMSI = Total of grades for all wall segments/# of wall segments analyzed

A score of 1.7 and above has been linked to a large area of infarction and worse prognosis [3].

Aortic dissection

Echocardiography is used extremely well in cases of a suspected aortic dissection. It may be used even when the patient is too unstable to have CT/MRI. The proximal ascending aorta is easily visualized on standard transthoracic echocardiography (TTE).

The distal ascending aorta, the aortic arch, and proximal descending aorta are best visualized by transesophageal echocardiography (TEE). There is a blind spot on the TEE and the distal part of the ascending aorta is usually not visualized due to attenuation from the air present in the trachea [4]. Multiple images, in multiple different views/angles of the aorta, must be analyzed prior to drawing conclusions about aortic dissection from echocardiography. Color Doppler interrogation of flow in the aorta is extremely important in this type of study. Clues towards the presence of an aortic dissection are [3]:

- An intimal flap, usually mobile, within the aorta (Figure 13.4).
- Color Doppler flow absent from specific parts of the aorta, and normal, pulsatile flow in other parts of the aorta.

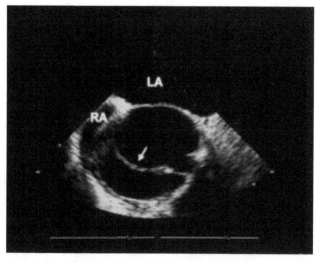

Figure 13.4 Aortic dissection flap (arrow), identifying an aortic dissection (Reproduced from Song *et al.* [5], with permission from Elsevier).

TTE has a sensitivity and specificity of approximately 70–80% to diagnose an aortic dissection. TEE has a sensitivity of 95–100% and a specificity 90–100% to diagnose an aortic dissection that is present in the area of the aorta that can be imaged (not below the level of the stomach). A more detailed discussion of aortic dissection is given in Chapter 8.

Pulmonary embolus

It is extremely difficult to visualize an actual thrombus on echocardiography, unless a large embolus is present in the RV outflow view in the pulmonary artery (Figure 13.5). Hemodynamic changes caused by a pulmonary embolus on the pulmonary artery and the right ventricle can easily be documented on a routine echocardiogram, although these are nonspecific.

In an acute PE, some of the possible echocardiographic signs are:
- Right ventricular dilatation (RVEDD >27 mm).
- RV free wall becomes hypokinetic.
- McConnell Sign (Figure 13.6) is highly suggestive of the presence of a pulmonary embolus [7].
- The pulmonary artery systolic pressure is usually elevated (TR velocity above 2.6 m/s). The pulmonary artery is also noted to be dilated (based on CT studies, 32.6 mm is the upper limit of normal diameter of the main pulmonary artery [9]). There is a loss of the respiratory-phasic collapse of the IVC.

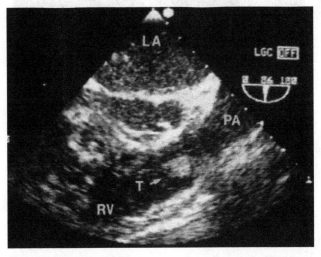

Figure 13.5 A thrombus (T) is noted in the right ventricle (RV) heading toward the pulmonary artery (PA) [6].

(a)

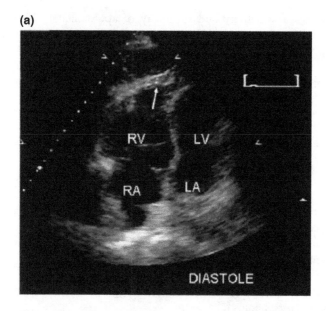

(b)

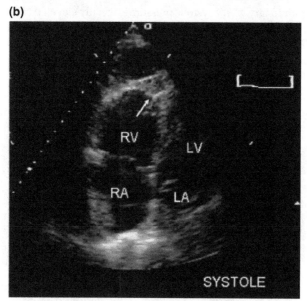

Figure 13.6 McConnell Sign. The RV apex [arrow in **(a)**] is seen clearly contracting in systole [arrow in **(b)**], while the free wall of the right ventricle is hypokinetic (Reproduced from Casazza *et al.* [8], with permission from Elsevier).

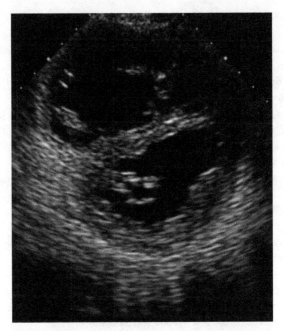

Figure 13.7 The LV in this systolic frame takes on a shape of a "D", indicating increased RV systolic pressure.

- The presence of the "60/60" sign (discussed in Chapter 8).
- RV pressure overload pattern with the "D-sign" (Figure 13.7, Chapter 8).
- RV/LV EDD ratio >0.7 [10].

With sensitivities and specificities for all of these echocardiographic findings to diagnose PE varying largely among multiple studies, it is clear that these findings can be used to aid in the diagnosis of a pulmonary embolus, but they cannot definitively establish such a diagnosis.

Other causes

It is important to note that many other causes of chest pain exist and that an echocardiogram is sometimes able to help in making such diagnoses. The more common causes are:

- Pericarditis – the presence of a small pericardial effusion can point toward the presence of acute pericarditis. However, the absence of an effusion does not rule out this diagnosis.

- Pleural effusion – the presence of a pleural effusion is sometimes noted on an echocardiogram (usually seen distal to the aorta on parasternal long and outside of the pericardium on apical images). Small or large pleural effusions are capable of causing chest pain.
- Musculoskeletal pain – no findings associated with echocardiography.
- GI-related symptoms – no findings associated with echocardiography.
- Masses – although rare, masses can be noted within and outside of the heart.

Due to the ease, speed, and noninvasive nature of an echocardiogram, it is widely utilized in patients who present with chest pain.

When faced with a patient with chest pain, it is necessary to make sure you:

- Check the parasternal and apical views, and analyze the motion of all myocardial segments.
- Analyze the RV free wall and apical motion to help in the diagnosis of pulmonary embolism.
- Look for RV volume and/or pressure overload pattern in the parasternal short axis views.
- Check all of the views of the ascending, transverse, and descending/abdominal aorta to look for aortic dissection.
- Always check for the presence of a pericardial effusion.

An echocardiogram can help guide the decision making process and speed up the diagnostic process of chest pain, therefore assuring the quick and appropriate delivery of treatment for patients with this clinical presentation.

References

1 Kimura BJ, Bocchicchio M, Willis CL, Demaria AN. Screening cardiac ultrasonographic examination in patients with suspected cardiac disease in the emergency department. *Am Heart J* 2001; 142(2):324–30.
2 Lang RM, Bierig M, Devereux RB, *et al*. Recommendations for Chamber Quantification: A Report from the American Society of Echocardiography's Guidelines and Standards Committee and the Chamber Quantification Writing Group, Developed in Conjunction with the European Association of Echocardiography, a Branch of the European Society of Cardiology. *J Am Soc Echocardiogr* 2005; 18(12):1440–63.
3 Galasko G, Basu S, Lahiri A, Senior R. A prospective comparison of echocardiographic wall motion score index and radionuclide ejection fraction in predicting outcome following acute myocardial infarction. *Heart* 2001; 86(3):271–76.
4 Shiga T, Wajima Z, Apfel CC, *et al*. Diagnostic accuracy of transesophageal echocardiography, helical computed tomography, and magnetic resonance imaging for suspected thoracic aortic dissection: systematic review and meta-analysis. *Arch Intern Med* 2006; 166(13):1350–6.

5 Song JK, Kim HS, Kang DH, *et al*. Different clinical features of aortic intramural hematoma versus dissection involving the ascending aorta. *J Am Coll Cardiol* 2001; 37(6):1604–10.

6 Van der Wouw PA, Koster RW, Delemarre BJ, *et al*. Diagnostic accuracy of transesophageal echocardiography during cardiopulmonary resuscitation. *J Am Coll Cardiol* 1997; 30(3):780–3.

7 Kurzyna M, Torbicki A, Pruszczyk P, *et al*. Disturbed right ventricular ejection pattern as a new Doppler echocardiographic sign of acute pulmonary embolism. *Am J Cardiol* 2002; 90(5):507–11.

8 Casazza F, Bongarzoni A, Capozi A, Agostoni O. Regional right ventricular dysfunction in acute pulmonary embolism and right ventricular infarction. *Eur J Echocardiogr* 2005; 6(1):11–4.

9 Karazincir S, Balci A, Seyfeli E, *et al*. CT assessment of main pulmonary artery diameter. *Diagn Interv Radiol* 2008; 14(2):72–4.

10 Kasper W, Meinertz T, Henkel B, *et al*. Echocardiographic findings in patients with proved pulmonary embolism. *Am Heart J* 1986; 112(6):1284–90.

Cardiac causes of syncope and acute neurological events

Erika R. Gehrie

Preferred Health Partners, New York, NY, USA

Syncope is a common neurological problem encountered by both the Emergency Room physician and the cardiologist. About 3% of all ER visits and 6% of all hospital admissions are for syncope. If the patient has known cardiac disease the likelihood that the event was cardiac in nature increases from 6.5 to 26.7% in men and from 3.8 to 16.8% in women [1]. The percentage of each cause of syncope in the Framingham Heart Study is shown in Table 14.1. Often a good history, physical exam and EKG will lead one to a diagnosis. The echocardiogram often confirms a suspected diagnosis and can rule out some potentially dangerous causes of syncope. (Table 14.1) [2].

Echocardiography is an extremely important tool in the diagnostic evaluation of patients with syncope. It is especially important with patients who have:
- known cardiovascular disease
- abnormal ECG

In these patients, an abnormal echocardiogram (EF <40%) points toward the diagnosis of arrhythmia, and a normal echocardiogram points toward noncardiac causes [2].

There are multiple causes of syncope and based on the suspected cause of the clinical presentation, specific echocardiographic measurements should be performed. These measurements are described here categorized by possible causes of syncope.

Practical Manual of Echocardiography in the Urgent Setting, First Edition.
Edited by Vladimir Fridman and Mario J. Garcia.
© 2013 John Wiley & Sons, Ltd. Published 2013 by John Wiley & Sons, Ltd.

Table 14.1 Causes of syncope (all values as %).	
Cardiac	9.5
Unknown	36.6
Stroke or TIA	4.1
Seizure	4.9
Vasovagal	21.2
Orthostatic	9.4
Medication	6.8
Other (cough syncope, situational syncope, micturition syncope)	7.5

Hypovolemia

- The focus in these patients is to establish the presence of a normal LV function and no major chamber size or valvular abnormalities.
- An echocardiogram can show a hyperdynamic and underfilled left ventricle.
- Occasionally an intracavity gradient can be detected (when PW Doppler volume is placed within the LV cavity and moved from apical portion to the base).
- Stroke volume, as calculated by methods explained in prior chapters, is important in these cases.
- A normal stroke volume is 70 ml. In these cases, the TVI of the valve (whichever one is chosen) suggests a low stroke volume, but is balanced by the tachycardia that is usually present in these patients.

Arrhythmias

This is a critical rule-out diagnosis for patients with syncope. Arrhythmias that can cause syncope range from simple supraventricular tachycardia to ventricular tachycardia/fibrillation. Short of actually recording an arrhythmic episode during an echocardiogram on the rhythm strip, the best way to predict arrhythmogenic potential of a patient is to evaluate for the presence of structural abnormalities.

Ischemic heart disease

Ventricular tachycardia related to a scar from a prior myocardial infarction.
- Regional wall motion abnormalities would hint toward the presence of a prior myocardial infarction and scar tissue which is a source of ventricular arrhythmias.

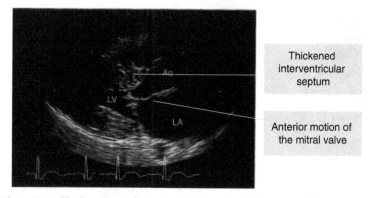

Figure 14.1 Thickened septum and anterior motion of the mitral valve in systole indicative of hypertrophic obstructive cardiomyopathy (Reproduced from Covington and Byrd [3]).

Dilated cardiomyopathy

- Ventricular tachycardia (VT) can occur in cardiomyopathies of any etiology.
- Evaluating overall ejection fraction with specific quantitative methods (as described in Chapter 4) is extremely important in syncope patients, since a lower EF increases the probability of ventricular tachycardia and fibrillation
- Regional wall motion abnormalities may be seen in regional myocarditis and sarcoid cardiomyopathy and increase the likelihood of VT.

Hypertrophic obstructive cardiomyopathy (HOCM)

- Myocardial hypertrophy, fibrosis and myocyte disarray all predispose a patient with HOCM to ventricular tachycardia and fibrillation.
- On echocardiography, increased septal thickness is a predictor of arrhythmia (Figure 14.1).
- The presence of systolic anterior motion (SAM) of the anterior mitral leaflet, which can cause acute left ventricular outflow obstruction, should be investigated (Figure 14.2).

RV-related arrhythmia

- Arrythmogenic right ventricular dysplasia (ARVD) is characterized by fatty tissue deposits, wall thinning and fibrosis in the right ventricle. This can lead to ventricular arrhythmias and syncope
- On echocardiography, RV dilatation and reduced function are major diagnostic criteria.
- RV regional wall motion abnormalities may be seen

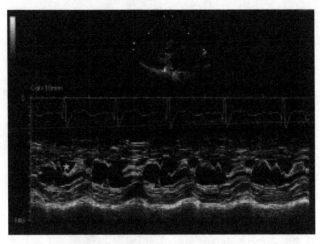

Figure 14.2 M-mode image of a patient with HOCM, showing anterior motion of the mitral valve in systole (asterisk) (Reproduced from Covington and Byrd [3]).

Aortic stenosis

- Syncope is one of the three symptoms which indicate a poorer prognosis in patients with aortic stenosis (syncope, heart failure, angina).
- A careful evaluation of the aortic valve (using the methods discussed in Chapter 5) must be undertaken in all syncope cases.

Cardiac tamponade

- Although rare, it must be considered in cases of syncope.
- Complete echocardiographic evaluation of tamponade is described in Chapter 9.

Pacemaker malfunction

- The only possible cause of pacemaker malfunction that can be evaluated with echocardiography is perforation/tamponade.
- Perforation of the pacemaker wire into the pericardial space is often accompanied by a localized effusion.

Endocarditis

- Endocarditis can be associated with complete heart block. An abscess involving the septal wall in aortic valve endocarditis is the most common finding.
- Full endocarditis evaluation is discussed in Chapter 17.

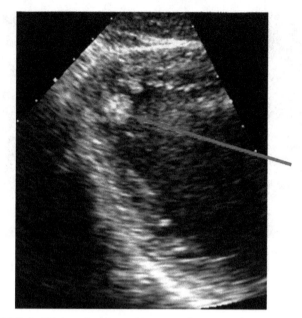

Figure 14.3 An LV thrombus (arrow) is seen at the apex of the left ventricle.

Pulmonary embolism

- Acute dilatation and dysfunction of the right ventricle and pulmonary hypertension should raise suspicion of the diagnosis.
- Full evaluation of PE cases is discussed in earlier chapters.

Stroke and transient ischemic attacks

Although most commonly the echocardiogram is normal or shows nonspecific abnormalities, it is extremely important to identify any possible cardiac cause of CVA/TIAs. In most cases the echocardiogram does not need to be performed urgently, unless critically needed to initiate anticoagulation.

The main objective is to rule out any possible causes of embolic phenomenon from the heart. Possibilities include:

- LV thrombus (Figure 14.3).
- Left atrial appendage thrombus – usually seen on a TEE (Figure 14.4)
  - It is important to differentiate left atrial appendage thrombus from normal structures in the left atrial appendage (such as pectinate muscle (Figure 14.5)) or nearby "Coumadin Ridge" (Figure 14.6).
  - Presence of "smoke", which is spontaneous echo contrast, has been shown to have thrombotic potential (Figure 14.6).

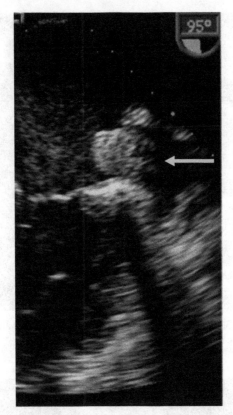

Figure 14.4 A large thrombus (arrow) is noted in the left atrial appendage.

- Aortic plaques (Figure 14.7) – the presence of plaques >4 mm in length has been shown to increase the risk of stroke in patients [5].
- PFO/ASD
  ○ Patent foramen ovale (PFO) can be diagnosed on TTE (subcostal view is best), or TEE (bicaval view). Sometimes, color Doppler alone is enough to visualize the defect (Figure 14.8). A TTE with agitated saline contrast can be performed, with imaging done in either apical or subcostal views, to more definitely check for a PFO (Figure 14.9).
  ○ Atrial septal defect (ASD) is important to diagnose if present. TEE is the best method to diagnose the presence of an ASD, and to determine the ASD type. Figure 14.10 shows an ostium secundum ASD, as seen in a bicaval view on a TEE.
- Interatrial septal aneurysm (IAS) is defined as excursion of interatrial septum >15 mm from the interatrial line: The significance of its presence to a patient is still debated. However, the presence of IAS

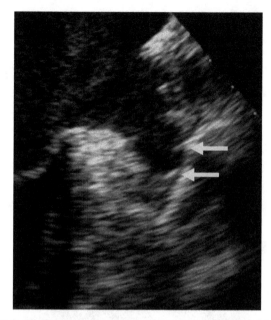

Figure 14.5 Small "finger-like" projections (arrows) into the left atrial appendage are pectinate muscles and are not thrombi.

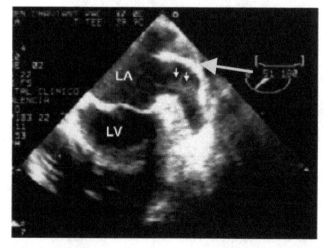

Figure 14.6 Spontaneous echo contrast is seen in the left atrial appendage (white arrows). The origin of the arrows is next to a normal structure that separates the left atrial appendage from the left superior pulmonary vein knows as the "Coumadin Ridge" (yellow arrow) [4].

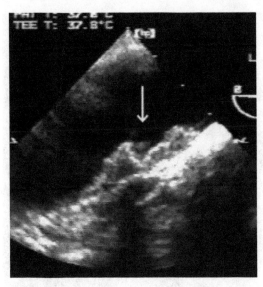

Figure 14.7 TEE view of the aorta shows a large atheromatous plaque (arrow) (Reproduced from Di Tullio *et al.* [5], with permission from Elsevier).

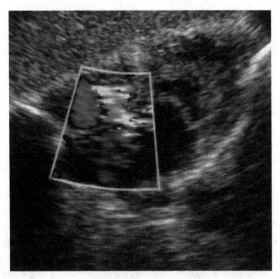

Figure 14.8 Color doppler of subcostal view shows flow between the right atrium and the left atrium, consistent with PFO or ASD.

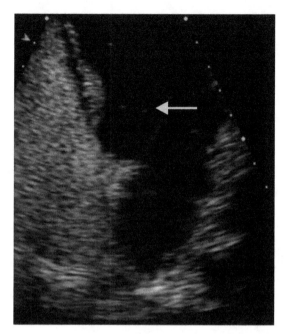

Figure 14.9 Presence of "bubbles" in the left heart chambers (arrow) after injection of agitated saline contrast into a vein indicates present of shunt, in this case a PFO.

with a PFO/ASD should be checked for, and noted, as it carries an increased embolic potential (Figure 14.11) [6, 7].

Cardiac masses [8]

Cardiac masses can cause neurological events, as they can form thrombi on their surface which can embolize, or they can cause obstructive valvular physiology when they grow to a large size.

- The most common cardiac tumors that carry an increased risk of embolization are:
  - Myxoma (Figure 14.12) – the most common primary tumor – usually are located attached to the interatrial septum, near the fossa ovalis.
  - Papillary fibroelastoma (Figure 14.13) – most common tumor of intracardiac valves. Described as having multiple small projections – "sea anemone" appearance.

When evaluating a patient for any neurological symptoms, cardiac causes of such symptoms should always be considered, and an echocardiogram should be performed in almost every case. A TTE should be

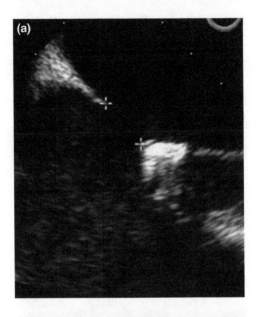

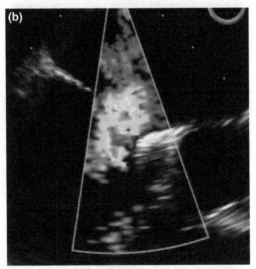

Figure 14.10 **(a)** The presence of an empty break (outlined by crosses) in the interatrial septum indicates the presence of an ASD. The location of this break determines what type of ASD is present, in this case ostium secundum ASD. **(b)** Color Doppler shows flow going through the ASD.

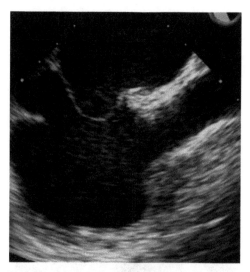

Figure 14.11 Clear inteatrial septal aneurysm is present in this TEE bicaval view.

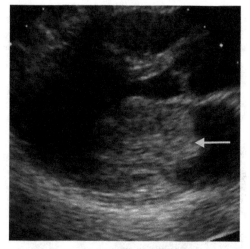

Figure 14.12 A large mass (arrow), later determined to be a myxoma, is seen in the left atrium, protruding into the left ventricle. Such a mass can cause cardiogenic shock due to its obstruction of the mitral valve inflow.

performed first, as a positive TTE finding will make a TEE unnecessary, thus sparing a patient from an invasive procedure. However, if a TTE does not help in determining the cardiac cause of a neurological event, a TEE should be considered. If the decision of the cardiology

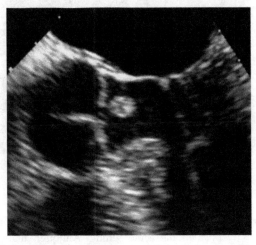

Figure 14.13 A mass on the aortic valve was shown to be a papillary fibroelastoma on a histology analysis.

and neurology teams taking care of the patient is to proceed with the TEE, it should be performed in a timely fashion in order to not delay the diagnosis and treatment of the patient.

References

1 Soteriades ES, Evans JC, Larson MG, *et al*. Incidence and prognosis of syncope. *N Engl J Med* 2002; 347:878.

2 Sarasin FP, Junod AF, Carballo D, *et al*. Role of echocardiography in the evaluation of syncope: a prospective study. *Heart* 2002; 88:363.

3 Covington MK, Byrd III BF. Congenital heart disease in adults: echocardiographic evaluation of left and right ventricular outflow tract obstruction. *Prog Pediatr Cardiol* 2003; 17:9–19.

4 Martinez-Brotons A, Chorro FJ, Insa L. An unusual cause of enhancement of the swirling motion of left atrial spontaneous echo contrast. *Int J Cardiol* 2003; 89(1):95–6.

5 Di Tullio, MR, Homma S, Jin Z, Sacco RL. Aortic atherosclerosis, hypercoagulatibility, and stroke: The APRIS (Aortic Plaque and Risk of Ischemic Stroke) Study. *J Am Coll Cardiol* 2008; 52(10):855–61.

6 Mugge A, Daniel WG, Angermann C, *et al*. Atrial septal aneurysm in adult patients. *Circulation* 1995; 91:2785–92.

7 Mattioli AV, Aquilina M, Oldani A, *et al*. Atrial septal aneurysm as a cardioembolic source in adult patients with stroke and normal carotid arteries. *Eur Heart J* 2001; 22:261–8.

8 Oh JK, Seward JB, Tajik AJ. *The Echo Manual*. New York: Wolters Kluwer/ Lippincott, Williams & Wilkins, 2006.

Acute dyspnea and heart failure

Mariusz W. Wysoczanski

Cardiovascular Diseases, Beth Israel Medical Center, Albert Einstein College of Medicine, New York, NY, USA

CHAPTER 15

This chapter aims to make practical the echocardiographic approach to the evaluation of dyspnea in the acute setting. Although many causes of dyspnea are noncardiac related, it is important to know when it is. The echocardiogram is likely the single most useful test in evaluating the etiology of the patient's dyspnea, if it is cardiac related, because of its ability to assess hemodynamics, global systolic and diastolic function, regional wall motion abnormalities, valvular function and pericardial disease [1].

Echocardiogram in "heart failure"

An echocardiogram performed for symptoms of heart failure must answer these important clinical questions:
- Is it systolic or diastolic heart failure?
- Is it right-sided or left-sided heart failure?
- What are the cardiac filling pressures?

1 Pathologies that cause elevation of left chamber "filling" pressures and/or restrict adequate left ventricular stroke volume trigger dyspnea via left heart failure.
2 Restriction of adequate cardiac output through the pulmonary vascular tree is the likely cause of dyspnea in right heart failure.
3 The hemodynamic consequences of numerous triggers can lead to dyspnea.

Practical Manual of Echocardiography in the Urgent Setting, First Edition.
Edited by Vladimir Fridman and Mario J. Garcia.
© 2013 John Wiley & Sons, Ltd. Published 2013 by John Wiley & Sons, Ltd.

Systolic or diastolic heart failure?

The ACC/AHA heart failure guidelines assign a class 1 indication for echocardiographic assessment in heart failure [2, 3]. The echocardiogram must determine whether:

- LVEF is preserved or reduced;
- the structure of the LV is normal or abnormal;
- there are other structural abnormalities.

Chapter 4 provides thorough instruction into the assessment of the ejection fraction (EF), stroke volume, as well as grading diastolic function. The following points are useful highlights for this topic:

- Acquire endocardial excursion and myocardial thickening via any echo window that the patient's clinical status allows for.
- Quantify the ejection fraction if appropriate.
- Assess diastolic function.
- Rule out acute cardiac pathology such as tamponade.
- Note any obvious regional wall motion if ischemia is a possibility [4].

After full evaluation of the systolic and diastolic function is performed, it then can be inferred whether the patient is suffering from systolic and/or diastolic heart failure. Patients with systolic heart failure can also have diastolic heart failure, and actually have a worse clinical prognosis if this is the case.

Intracardiac pressures

- Echocardiography can be extremely helpful in estimating intracardiac pressures.
- Measurements are based on the Bernoulli equation where velocities are translated into pressure gradients [5]: Pressure gradient$=4(velocity)^2$.
- Diastolic measurements, as described in Chapter 4, hint at the left-sided filling pressures.

The following are validated echocardiographic interrogation techniques and values, listed with their respective chambers [6, 7].

Right atrial pressure

- As right atrial pressure (RAP) increases, and pressure is transmitted backwards, the inferior vena cava (IVC) dilates and resists normal inspiratory collapse.
- In subcostal view, rotate the probe towards the right shoulder until the junction of the IVC-RA is noted (Figure 15.1).
- The IVC diameter should be measured approximately 0.5–3.0 cm proximal to the entrance to the right atrium (RA) while it is perpendicular to the long axis, during end-expiration (Figure 15.1).

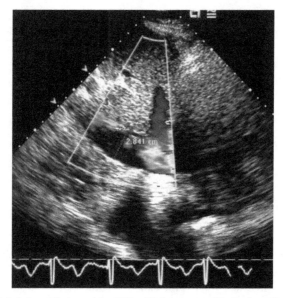

Figure 15.1 Subcostal view of the IVC with flow reversal in the hepatic vein by color Doppler (red signal). The plethoric IVC measures 2.8 cm. Both findings suggest markedly elevated RA pressures.

- Run the mentioned view live under 2D or by M-mode and assess for collapsibility during the normal respiratory cycle of the patient.
- Chapter 4 described values for RA pressures. However, a cutoff value of 2.1cm should be kept in mind.
- Hepatic vein flow:
  - At low or normal RAP, there is systolic predominance in hepatic vein flow, such that the velocity of the systolic wave (Vs) is greater than the velocity of the diastolic wave (Vd).
  - At elevated RAP, this systolic predominance is lost, such that Vs is substantially decreased and Vs/Vd is <1 and suggests a RAP of 15mm Hg.
  - This PW interrogation of the hepatic vein is done via the same subcostal window with the sample volume in a hepatic vein emptying into the IVC.
- It should be noted that in normal young athletes, the IVC may be dilated in the presence of normal pressure.

Right ventricular systolic pressure and systolic pulmonary artery pressure

- Right ventricular systolic pressure (RVSP) and systolic pulmonary artery pressure (SPAP) are used interchangeably in the absence of a right ventricular outflow tract or pulmonary valve gradient (i.e., pulmonary valve stenosis and congenital heart disease).

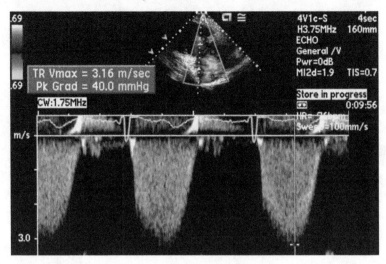

Figure 15.2 CW Doppler interrogation through the tricuspid valve yields the profile whose maximum velocity is 3.1 m/s. This translates into a gradient of 40 mm Hg, which is added to the right atrial pressure to estimate the SPAP.

- RVSP/SPAP can be reliably determined from peak tricuspid regurgitation (TR) jet velocity.
- $RVSP = 4V^2 + RAP$, where V is the peak velocity (in meters per second) of the TR jet and RAP is the estimated value described in the previous section (Figure 15.2).
- Interrogation of the TR velocities can be appreciated in the following views:
  - right ventricular inflow;
  - basal short axis;
  - apical four-chamber;
  - subcostal four-chamber;
- Note that the maximum TR velocity at any of these views represents the true velocity.
- To obtain TR velocity, it is necessary to:
  - visualize the tricuspid valve;
  - activate the color Doppler to appreciate the TR jet;
  - activate cursor and attempt to align the TR jet parallel to the sample volume;
  - activate the continuous wave (CW) Doppler;
  - freeze the TR Doppler jet profile while using a sweep speed of 100 mm/s;
  - record the peak TR velocity;
  - enhance the signal with agitated salineif it is weak.

Note that in patients with very severe TR (such that the leaflets do not coapt), the Doppler envelope may be cut off because of an early equalization of RVSP and RAP, and the simplified Bernoulli equation may underestimate the true RV–RA gradient.

LV filling pressures

The American Society of Echocardiography (ASE) has stated that the assessment of LV filling pressures should be split into two groups based upon the EF [8].

In patients with depressed EF (Figure 15.3):

- E/A <1 suggests normal filling pressures.
- E/A >2 suggests elevated filling pressures.
- E/A of 1–2 is indeterminate and requires further differentiation such that:
  o average E/e′ <8 suggest normal filling pressures;
  o average E/e′ >15 suggest elevated filling pressures;

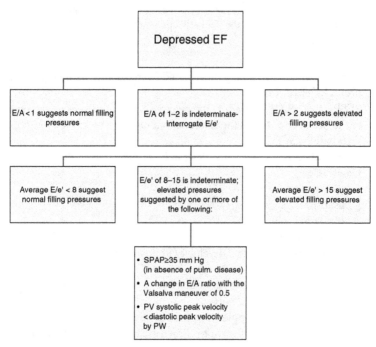

Figure 15.3 Diagnostic algorithm for the estimation of left ventricular filling pressures in patients with depressed ejection fraction. EF: ejection fraction; E: early mitral inflow velocity; A: late mitral inflow velocity; e′: early annular diastolic velocity; SPAP: systolic pulmonary artery pressure; pulm: pulmonary; PV: pulmonary vein; PW: pulsed wave Doppler.

o E/e′ of 8–15 is indeterminate; elevated pressures are suggested by one or more:
- SPAP ≥35 mm Hg (in absence of pulmonary disease);
- a change in E/A ratio with the Valsalva maneuver of 0.5;
- systolic peak velocity/diastolic peak velocity ratio in pulmonary venous flow of <1 measured by PW Doppler.

In patients with normal EF (Figure 15.4):
- E/e′ ≤8 at either annulus suggest normal filling pressures.
- Average E/e′ ≥13 suggest elevated filling pressures (≥12 lat and ≥15 sep annulus).
- E/e′ of 9–12 is indeterminate; elevated pressures are suggested by any of the following:
  o SPAP ≥35 mm Hg (in absence of pulmonary disease);
  o a change in E/A ratio with the Valsalva maneuver of 0.5.
  o maximal LA volume ≥34 ml/m².

It is important to note that the E/e′ ratio is not accurate as an index of filling pressures in patients with heavy annular calcification and constrictive pericarditis. The latter should be suspected when the patient presents in predominant right heart failure, has a normal EF, and the tissue Doppler e′ is ≥8 cm/s.

An indicator of high LVEDP is the presence of a "B-bump" on M-mode echocardiography of the mitral valve (Figure 15.5). Although rarely seen, when is noted it is indicative of high LV filling pressures.

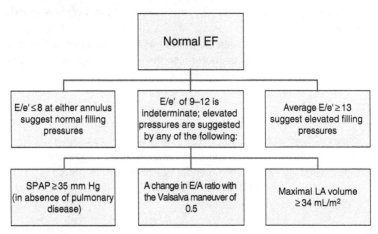

Figure 15.4 Diagnostic algorithm for the estimation of left ventricular filling pressures in patients with normal ejection fraction.

EF: ejection fraction; E: early mitral inflow velocity; A: late mitral inflow velocity; e′: early annular diastolic velocity; SPAP: systolic pulmonary artery pressure; LA: left atrium.

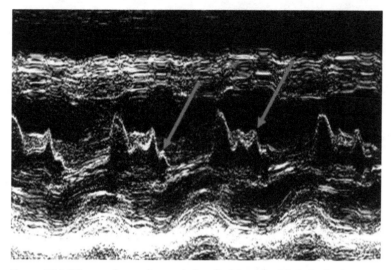

Figure 15.5 B-bumps (arrows) are noted on the M-mode of the mitral valve, indicative of high LV filling pressures.

Echocardiographic approach to dyspnea with hypoxemia

Hypoxemia can originate from the cardiovascular system via:
- Ventilation–perfusion (V/Q) mismatch, as seen in a pulmonary embolism (PE) or pulmonary hypertension (PH), and often responds to 100% O_2.
- Right-to-left shunting, seen in pulmonary edema, intracardiac and intrapulmonary shunts, is poorly responsive to O_2, and often requires positive end-expiratory pressure [9].

VQ mismatch
- A comprehensive evaluation of the cardiovascular causes of V/Q mismatch, including PE and PH, is provided in prior chapters.
- The hemodynamic profile consistent with these syndromes is:
  ○ decreased stroke volume secondary to restricted LV filling;
  ○ normal or reduced LV filling pressures;
  ○ elevated right chamber pressures.

Shunting
Pulmonary edema
- Results in hypoxemia by flooding the alveoli and reactive shunting.
- Elevated LVEDP or pulmonary capillary wedge pressures (PCWP) is the hallmark finding when a patient presents in heart failure.

Intracardiac and intrapulmonary shunting
- Multiple causes (as described in prior chapters).
- Can occur due to opening of a patent foramen ovale (PFO), with consequent right-to-left shunting [10].
- Contrast must be used to identify level of shunting if not detected by color Doppler.

Differential diagnosis for cardiac induced dyspnea

The specific cardiac lesion leading to acute dyspnea can be discovered by analyzing the five "V"s:
- Vessels
- Volts
- Ventricles
- Valves
- Volume.

Included under each of these are:
- Vessels: acute coronary syndrome, hypertensive crisis, pulmonary embolism, aortic dissection, pulmonary hypertension, intrapulmonary shunts.
- Volts: tachyarrhythmias, bradyarrhythmias.
- Ventricles: primary cardiomyopathy, decompensated systolic/diastolic heart failure, cardiac tamponade, constrictive pericarditis, intracardiac shunts, dynamic left ventricular outflow tract (LVOT) obstruction.
- Valves: acute valvular regurgitation (ruptured chordae/papillary muscle, infective endocarditis).
- Volume: fluid shift or fluid retention with acute fluid overload.

Algorithm for treatment

To properly treat the patient, it is necessary to establish:
- Is there evidence of compromise to the hemodynamics of the heart?
- What is the likely culprit responsible for the disturbance?

Figure 15.6 provides a systemic approach to this inquiry.
- Begin with an estimation of the ejection fraction and intracardiac pressures, as outlined earlier in this chapter.
- Look for clues in the differential diagnosis of the five "V"s. Remember that only what can be adequately interrogated can effectively be ruled out.
- Use the findings to aid in the clinical diagnosis as well as to guide therapy.

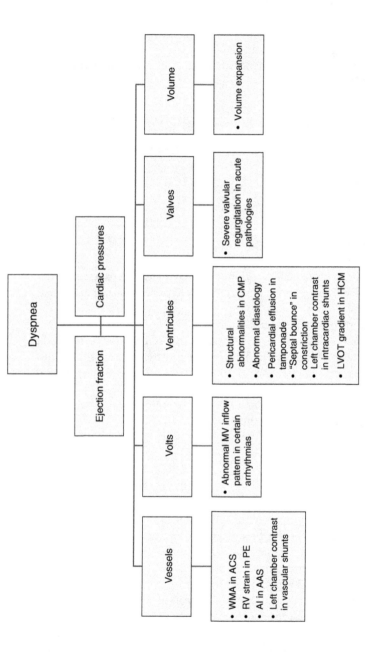

Figure 15.6 Algorithm for a practical echocardiographic approach to dyspnea in the acute setting. Evaluating ejection fraction and cardiac pressures gauges the extent of cardiovascular contribution to dyspnea followed by an assessment of the five elements for clues to the culprit lesion. WMA: wall motion abnormality; ACS: acute coronary syndrome; RV: right ventricle; PE: pulmonary embolism; AI: aortic insufficiency; AAS: acute aortic syndrome; CMP: cardiomyopathy; LVOT: left ventricular outflow tract; HCM: hypertrophic cardiomyopathy.

References

1 Libby P, Bonow RO, Mann DL, Zipes DP. *Braunwald's Heart Disease*, 8th edn. Philadelphia: Elsevier Publishing, 2008: 595.

2 Hunt SA, Abraham WT, Chin MH, *et al*. 2009 Focused update incorporated into the ACC/AHA 2005 guidelines for the diagnosis and management of heart failure in adults: a report of the American College of Cardiology Foundation/ American Heart Association Task Force on Practice Guidelines: developed in collaboration with the International Society for Heart and Lung Transplantation. *Circulation* 2009; 119(14):e391–e479.

3 Hunt SA, Abraham WT, Chin MH, *et al*. ACC/AHA 2005 Guideline update for the diagnosis and management of chronic heart failure in the adult: a report of the American College of Cardiology/American Heart Association Task Force on Practice Guidelines (Writing Committee to Update the 2001 Guidelines for the Evaluation and Management of Heart Failure). *Circulation* 2005; 112(12):e154–e235.

4 Lang RM, Bierig M, Devereux RB, *et al*. Recommendations for chamber quantification: a report from the American Society of Echocardiography's Guidelines and Standards Committee and the Chamber Quantification Writing Group, developed in conjunction with the European Association of Echocardiography, a branch of the European Society of Cardiology. *J Am Soc Echocardiogr* 2005; 18:1440–1463.

5 Armstrong WF, Ryan T. *Feigenbaum's Echocardiography*, 7th edn. Philadelphia: Lippincott, Williams & Wilkins, 2010: 212.

6 Oh JK, Seward JB, Tajik AJ. *The Echo Manual*, 3rd edn. Philadelphia: Lippincott, Williams & Wilkins, 2006: 81–82.

7 Rudski LG, Wyman WL, Afilalo J, *et al*. Guidelines for the echocardiographic assessment of the right heart in adults: a report from the American Society of Echocardiography endorsed by the European Association of Echocardiography, a registered branch of the European Society of Cardiology, and the Canadian Society of Echocardiography. *J Am Soc Echocardiogr* 2010; 23:685–713.

8 Nagueh SF, Appleton CP, Gillebert TC, *et al*. Recommendations for the evaluation of left ventricular diastolic function by echocardiography. *J Am Soc Echocardiogr* 2009; 22(2):107–133.

9 Kasper DL, Braunwald E, Fauci AS, *et al*, *Harrison's Principles of Internal Medicine*, 16th edn. New York: McGraw-Hill, 2005: 1501–1505.

10 Armstrong WF, Ryan T. *Feigenbaum's Echocardiography*, 7th edn. Philadelphia: Lippincott, Williams & Wilkins, 2010: 671.

Evaluation of a new heart murmur

Vinay Manoranjan Pai

Cardiovascular Diseases, Beth Israel Medical Center and Long Island College Hospital, New York, NY, USA

Mitral and aortic regurgitation are the more common valvular causes of a new heart murmur in the acute setting. Myxomatous degeneration, endocarditis and papillary muscle rupture are the common causes of acute mitral regurgitation whereas endocarditis is the common cause of acute aortic regurgitation. Ischemic mitral regurgitation following infarction or severe ischemia results more commonly from left ventricular remodeling and distortion of the mitral valve apparatus than papillary muscle rupture. Acute ventricular septal rupture is identified on Doppler echocardiography as a high velocity turbulent jet with a left-to-right shunt. Echocardiography should be performed in patients with peri-infarct pericardial rub to detect the presence of pericardial effusion.

Acute valvular regurgitation

Acute severe valvular regurgitation has a varied presentation and its early detection by accurate history, examination and diagnostic techniques can be life saving. Mitral and aortic regurgitation are the more common valvular causes of a new heart murmur in the acute setting. Echocardiography can be used not only in the diagnosis and severity of the condition but also in its mechanisms and etiologies.

- Common causes of acute native valve mitral regurgitation [1]:
  - Flail leaflet due to myxomatous degeneration (mitral valve prolapse), infective endocarditis, or trauma.
  - Ruptured chordae tendinae due to infective endocarditis, idiopathic (spontaneous) rupture, acute rheumatic fever or trauma (Figures 16.1 and 16.2).

Practical Manual of Echocardiography in the Urgent Setting, First Edition.
Edited by Vladimir Fridman and Mario J. Garcia.
© 2013 John Wiley & Sons, Ltd. Published 2013 by John Wiley & Sons, Ltd.

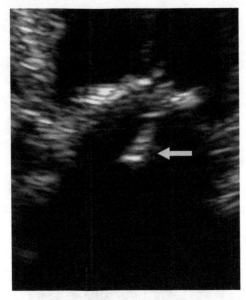

Figure 16.1 Rupture of mitral valve chordae as noted on an apical four-chamber view. The chordae is noted flailing (arrow) into the left atrium in this systolic frame.

- Papillary muscle rupture due to acute myocardial infarction or severe ischemia or trauma.
- Common causes of acute native valve aortic regurgitation:
  - Infective endocarditis causing leaflet perforation or destruction.
  - Aortic dissection.
  - Trauma.
- Causes of acute prosthetic valve regurgitation [2]:
  - Tissue valve leaflet rupture due to degeneration, calcification, or endocarditis.
  - Impaired closure of mechanical valve occluders due to valve thrombosis, infection, or pannus formation.
  - Paravalvular regurgitation due to infection or suture rupture.
- Acute mitral regurgitation (MR) due to endocarditis:
  - May result from leaflet perforation and ruptured chordae leading to the development of new heart murmurs.
  - If the infection extends to the adjoining annular tissue, a paravalvular abscess may be seen.
- Acute MR due to ruptured chordae tendinae (Figures 16.1 and 16.2):
  - Chordae tendinae can rupture spontaneously or may be the result of:
    - myxomatous degeneration as seen in mitral valve prolapse;

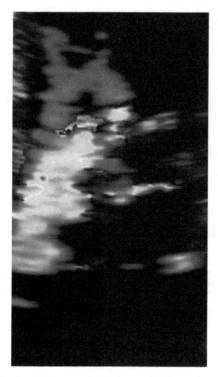

Figure 16.2 Moderate mitral regurgitation is noted in the patient from Figure 16.1.

- infective endocarditis;
- acute rheumatic fever.
  - The number of chordae involved and the rate of rupture determine acuity and severity of MR [1].
  - Anterior mitral valve leaflet chordal rupture is more frequently associated with rheumatic mitral valve disease, whereas posterior leaflet chordae were affected in mitral valve prolapse [3]. In the latter, ruptured chordae may or may not be accompanied by annular dilatation [4]
- Acute MR due to coronary artery disease:
  - Ischemic mitral regurgitation following infarction or severe ischemia results from:
    - left ventricular remodeling;
    - distortion of the mitral valve apparatus [5];
    - papillary muscle disruption is possible, and is a more dramatic and serious complication requiring urgent intervention.
  - In inferior/posterior MI the regurgitation jet is eccentric and posteriorly oriented [6] (Figure 16.3).

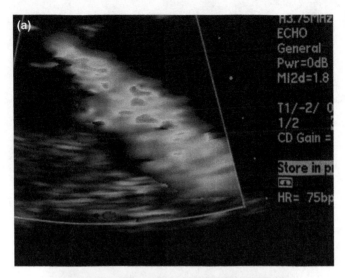

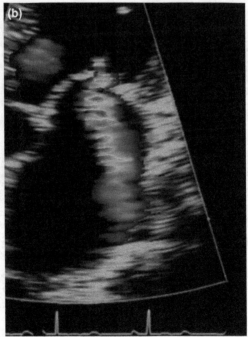

Figure 16.3 Inferiorly and posteriorly directed mitral regurgitation jet in a patient with history of RCA disease is seen in the **(a)** parasternal long and **(b)** apical five-chamber views.

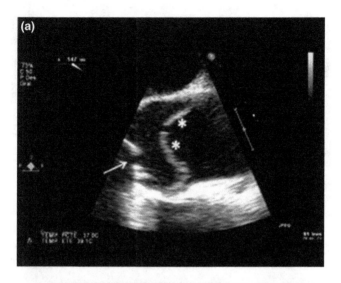

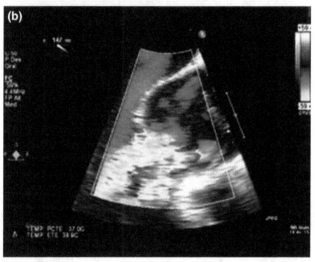

Figure 16.4 (a) A dissection flap (asterisk) is noted in the ascending aorta with malcoaptation of the aortic leafleats (arrow). **(b)** Severe aortic regurgitation is noted on color doppler in this patient (Reproduced from Fernandez-Jimenez *et al*. [7], with permisison from Elsevier).

- Posteriomedial papillary muscle, which is supplied by the right coronary artery, is more frequently involved as compared to the anterolateral one, which has dual blood supply: left circumflex and the left anterior descending.

- o Since both the anterior and posterior leaflets are supported by the posterior papillary muscle, inferior infarction can result in regurgitation through any of the mitral valve leaflets.
- Acute MR due to trauma:
  - o Blunt chest trauma → Increased intracardiac pressure against closed mitral valve → Posterior leaflet tear from mitral annulus or annular dehiscence → Eccentric mitral regurgitation jet.
  - o Normal left ventricular size with either normal or hyperdynamic function should raise suspicion for the regurgitation to be acute in onset.
  - o Since the left-sided chambers have not had time to adapt to the acute MR, pulmonary edema, shock and/or biventricular failure develops.
- Acute AR due to aortic dissection (Figure 16.4):
  - o In aortic dissection, acute AR results from annular or aortic root dilatation leading to incomplete coaptation of the valve leaflets or extension of the dissection into the valve itself.
  - o Due to the acuity of the situation, the left ventricle has no time to adapt to the volume overload leading to increase in the left ventricular end diastolic pressure, resulting in premature closure of the mitral valve and elevated left atrial and pulmonary venous pressures, ultimately leading to pulmonary edema.
  - o Inability of the left ventricle to increase the stroke volume leads to hypotension and shock.

Intracardiac shunts

Ventricular septal rupture is a rare but life threatening complication occurring in the first week after myocardial infarction resulting in cardiogenic shock.

- It is more frequently associated with anterior than other types of acute myocardial infarction.
- It is clinically diagnosed by the appearance of new harsh systolic murmur accompanied by hemodynamic deterioration, differential diagnosis of which is acute MR.
- Diagnostic imaging modality of choice is Doppler echocardiography (Figure 16.5).
- Rupture is identified by visualization of a high velocity turbulent jet with a left-to-right shunt.
- Echocardiography can also pinpoint the site and size of ventricular septal rupture, left and right ventricular function, and estimated right ventricular systolic pressure [9].

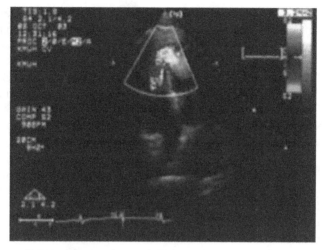

Figure 16.5 Color Doppler in an apical four-chamber view showing a ventricular septal defect involving the apical septum (Reproduced from Su *et al.* [8], with permisison from Elsevier)

Pericardial effusion

- Can be associated with a pericardial friction rub.
- Multiple possible etiologies (as described in Chapter 9).
- Echocardiography should be performed in such patients for a full analysis of hemodynamics (as described in Chapter 9).

Post myocardial infarction

Any new murmur (or any new chest pain, shortness of breath, heart failure) post myocardial infarction warrants an emergent echocardiogram for the evaluation of the following mechanical complications of MI:
- Ventricular free wall rupture
- Ventricular septal rupture
- Papillary muscle rupture or chordae tendinae rupture with acute mitral regurgitation
- Formation/rupture of LV pseudoaneurysm
- Formation of LV aneurysm
- Right ventricular failure
- Dynamic LVOT obstruction (a rare complication of MI).

In general, acute murmurs, especially with new symptoms, warrant speedy evaluation of the new findings. Most of the time, this involves an urgent, comprehensive, echocardiographic examination to determine the cause of the murmur. Once the diagnosis has been established, treatment can begin and, in many of these clinical situations, can be lifesaving.

References

1 Otto CM, Bonow RO. Valvular Heart disease: mitral regurgitation. In: Libby P, Bonow RO, Mann DL, Zipes DP (eds) *Braunwald's Heart Disease*, 8th Edition. Philadelphia: Saunders, 2007, 1657–69.

2 Otto, CM. Pathophysiology, clinical features, and management of acute mitral regurgitation. http://www.uptodate.com/contents/pathophysiology-clinical-features-and-management-of-acute-mitral-regurgitation (accessed November 17, 2012).

3 Kaymaz C, Ozdemir N, Ozkan M. Differentiating clinical and chocardiographic characteristics of chordal rupture detected in patients with rheumatic mitral valve disease and floppy mitral valve: impact of the infective endocarditis on chordal rupture. *Eur J Echocardiogr* 2005; 6(2):117–26.

4 Roberts WC, McIntosh CL, Wallace RB. Mechanisms of severe mitral regurgitation in mitral valve prolapse determined from analysis of operatively excised valves. *Am Heart J* 1987; 113(5):1316–23.

5 Bursi F, Enriquez-Sarano M, Jacobsen SJ, Roger VL. Mitral regurgitation after myocardial infarction: a review. *Am J Med* 2006; 119:103–12.

6 Chenzbraun, A. Echocardiography in acute chest pain and coronary syndromes: mechanical complications of AMI. In: Chenzbraun A (ed.) *Emergency Echocardiography*. Springer, 2009, 87–101.

7 Fernandez-Jimenez R, Vivas D, de Agustín JA, *et al.* Acute aortic dissection with ongoing right coronary artery and aortic involvement. *Int J Cardiol* 2012; 161(2):e34–6.

8 Su HM, Voon WC, Lin CC, *et al.* Ventricular septal rupture after early successful thrombolytic therapy in acute myocardial infarction: a case report. *Kaohsiung J Med Sci* 2004; 20:235–9.

9 Birnbaum Y, Fishbein MC, Blanche C, Siegel RJ. Ventricular septal rupture after acute myocardial infarction. *N Engl J Med* 2002; 347(18):1426–32.

Infective endocarditis

Luis Aybar

Cardiovascular Diseases, Beth Israel Medical Center, New York, NY, USA

CHAPTER 17

Since 1885, when Osler first made observations regarding infective endocarditis, important advances have been made in its diagnostic evaluation and management [1, 2, 3]. Morbidity and mortality of endocarditis remain high, making it one of the most catastrophic infectious and cardiac disease processes.

- In-hospital mortality rates of 15–20%.
- One-year mortality of up to 40% [4, 5].

Early diagnosis and treatment greatly increase the chance of successful outcome [6]. Echocardiography is the gold standard diagnostic test [7].

Diagnosis and diagnostic accuracy

- Infective endocarditis is diagnosed on the basis of multiple findings rather than a single definitive test [8].
- The modified Duke criteria, which are based on major and minor criteria, are used to label the diagnosis as "definitive", "possible" or "rejected" infective endocarditis (Figure 17.1) [8].
- Positive echocardiography is one of the major criteria for endocarditis.
- Sensitivity of TTE: 65–80%; Specificity of TTE: >90%.
- The chance of a false negative study is greatly increased by:
  - presence of pre-existing structural changes (e.g., prosthetic valves, degenerative valvular lesions, mitral valve prolapse, etc.) [9];
  - presence of nonoscillating or very small vegetations [10].
- Sensitivity of TEE: 95%; Specificity of TEE >90% [11, 12].

Practical Manual of Echocardiography in the Urgent Setting, First Edition.
Edited by Vladimir Fridman and Mario J. Garcia.
© 2013 John Wiley & Sons, Ltd. Published 2013 by John Wiley & Sons, Ltd.

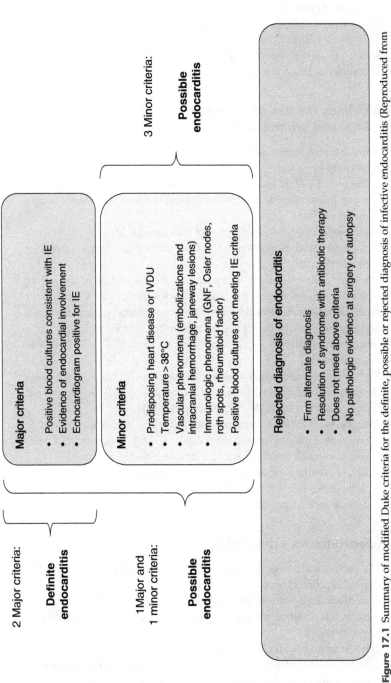

Figure 17.1 Summary of modified Duke criteria for the definite, possible or rejected diagnosis of infective endocarditis (Reproduced from Li *et al.* [8L with permission from OUP).

IE: Infective Endocarditis; IVDU: Intravenous drug use; GNF: Glomerulo-nephritis

- Cases have been described of negative TEEs early in the disease course but subsequent TEEs showing positive findings [13].
- If there is a high clinical suspicion of endocarditis with a negative initial TEE, it may be reasonable to repeat a TEE in 7–10 days. Further repetition carries a very low diagnostic utility (14).

Guidelines for use of echocardiography to diagnose endocarditis

- The American Society of Echocardiography assigns the highest appropriateness score to:
  - o the use of TTE to evaluate a case of suspected native or prosthetic valve infective endocarditis with positive blood cultures or a new murmur;
  - o to re-evaluate a case of diagnosed endocarditis at high risk for progression or complication or with a change in clinical status or physical exam.
- These guidelines consider inappropriate the use of TTE in the setting of transient fever without evidence of bacteremia or a new murmur or when bacteremia is caused by a pathogen not typically associated with endocarditis and/or the source is clearly not endovascular.
- Routine surveillance of uncomplicated endocarditis by TTE is also discouraged [7].
- Earlier guidelines for management of valvular disease placed a Class IIb (less well established evidence) on the use of TTE for any patient with nosocomial staphylococcal bacteremia [15].
- TEE use as an initial or supplemental test is accepted when there is:
  - o moderate to high pretest probability (e.g., staph bacteremia, fungemia, prosthetic heart valve, or intracardiac device);
  - o TTE is nondiagnostic due to poor imaging quality [7];
  - o Some have suggested that TEE be used or considered for every patient with suspected infective endocarditis.

Appearance on echocardiography

- The presence of a vegetation on a TTE or TEE must be evaluated in the individual clinical scenario [16].
- Noninfective vegetations should be in the differential diagnosis.
- Intracardiac masses are also important to separate from infective vegetations [9].
- Echocardiographic features of infective endocarditis include:
  - o an oscillating intracardiac mass on a valve, supporting structure or in the path of a regurgitant jet or an intracardiac device;

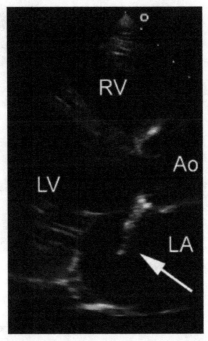

Figure 17.2 Vegetation (arrow) noted likely involving the mitral and aortic valves, as well as the intervalvular fibrosa (Reproduced from Bashore *et al.* [19], with permisison from Elsevier).

- ○ abscesses;
- ○ new partial dehiscence of a prosthetic valve;
- ○ new valvular regurgitation [17];
- ○ vegetations characteristically are echogenic masses attached to the valve, endocardial surface or prosthetic material and tend to be mobile, frequently showing high-frequency flutter or oscillations [18].
- The most commonly affected valves are the mitral and aortic valves (Figure 17.2).
- An intracardiac abscess is typically seen as a paravalvular echolucent zone with either no Doppler flow or Doppler flow in and out of the abscess (Figure 17.3) [19].
- Abscesses are more common in aortic valve endocarditis and frequently involve the tissue between the aortic and mitral valve [20].
- TTE is only 50% sensitive to intracardiac abscesses, while TEE increases sensitivity to 90% [21].
- TEE must be performed in any case for which there is a high clinical suspicion of abscess.

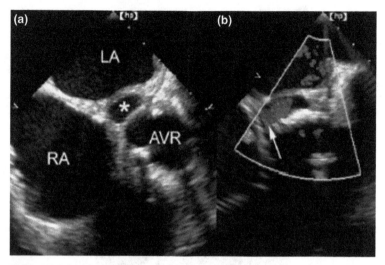

Figure 17.3 (a) Abscess formation near a prosthetic aortic valve (asterisk); (b) color Doppler shows flow (arrow) within the abscess (Reproduced from Bashore *et al.* [19], with permisison from Elsevier).

- A paravalvular echolucent zone that may or may not be pulsatile, with color Doppler flow inside, is usually a pseudoaneurysm. This can form a fistula [22].
- A dedicated cardiac CT has been shown to aid in the assessment of the paravalvular extent of abscess, pseudoaneurysms and fistulae [22].
- Valvular perforation can occur.
  ○ The anterior leaflet of the mitral valve is the most susceptible to perforation and typically occurs in the setting of aortic valve endocarditis and regurgitation.
  ○ Perforations are visualized as an interruption of valvular tissue traversed by color Doppler flow [9, 23].
- Saccular bulging of the anterior leaflet of the mitral valve into the left atrium is a valvular aneurysm, a less common complication of endocarditis that can lead to heart failure [9)].

Complications and risk stratification

Up to 35–40% of patients undergoing treatment for infective endocarditis will develop complications, the most frequent being heart failure, stroke and other forms of embolization and intracardiac abscess formation [6].
- Surgical intervention:
  ○ Life-threatening congestive heart failure due to severe valvular stenosis or regurgitation is the most common indication for surgery due to the high mortality associated [15].

- o Severe valvular regurgitation the presence of a normal left ventricular size is suggestive of an acute process, prompting surgery [24, 25].
- o Is indicated in elevated left ventricular end-diastolic or left atrial pressures and moderate-to-severe pulmonary hypertension [15].
- o Annular or aortic abscess and penetrating lesions (e.g., fistula between the Sinus of Valsalva and the right or left atria or right ventricle, mitral valve perforation with aortic valve endocarditis, infection in the annulus fibrosa) are other Class I indications for surgery [15].
- o Prosthetic valve involvement is not always an indication for surgery, unless presenting with heart failure, valve dehiscence, abscess formation or worsening regurgitation or obstruction [15].
- o Vegetation size >10 mm has been associated with a higher risk for embolization [26] and the combination of a size >15 mm with mobility confers an even greater risk [27, 28]. Surgical intervention on this basis alone remains controversial [15].

Prosthetic valve endocarditis

- Occurs in up to 1–6% of patients with valve prostheses [29, 30]
- Currently accounts for up to 30% of all cases of endocarditis.
- Has a higher frequency of abscesses and other paravalvular complications (Figures 17.3 and 17.4) [31].

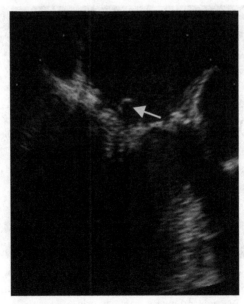

Figure 17.4 A vegetation is noted (arrow) attached to a prosthetic mitral valve.

- While there are similar rates of infective endocarditis among mechanical and bioprosthetic valves [31], there are basic differences in the appearance of complications:
  - o mechanical valves tend to have complications at the site of the junction between the sewing ring and the annulus, producing abscesses and dehiscence;
  - o bioprosthetic valves will more commonly have leaflet perforations and have a higher frequency of vegetations [32].
- If prosthetic valve endocarditis is considered, a TEE is usually necessary, especially in the setting mitral valve prosthesis.
- Frequently, the only echocardiographic finding of infective endocarditis will be paravalvular regurgitation or increased valvular regurgitation, when compared to baseline echocardiogram

Cardiac device-related infective endocarditis

- Incidence: 1.9 per 1000 device-years.
- Has considerable morbidity, mortality and cost [33, 34].
- On echocardiography, special attention must be given to:
  - o the tricuspid valve leaflets;
  - o entire device lead(s) including in the superior vena cava and the in right atrium;
  - o the endocardial wall (Figures 17.5 and 17.6).

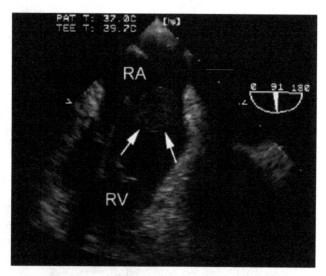

Figure 17.5 A vegetation resembling a ball (arrows) is noted attached to a cardiac rhythm device lead (Reproduced from Bashore *et al.* [19], with permisison from Elsevier). RA: right atrium; RV: right ventricle

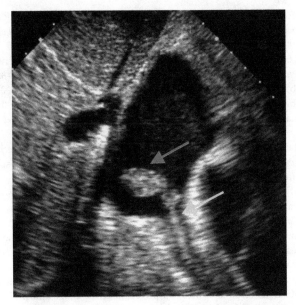

Figure 17.6 In this subcostal view, a vegetation (blue arrow) is noted attached to a cardiac rhythm device lead (yellow arrow) in the right atrium.

- TTE carries a poor sensitivity and negative predictive value and it is important to follow up a negative study with a TEE [35, 36].
- TEE must be done if diagnosis is considered, as management of device-related infective endocarditis requires removal of the device [34].
- If vegetation is >25 mm, surgical removal should be considered.
- Once device and lead extraction is performed a repeat echocardiogram should rule out residual infective lesions [35, 36].

References

1 Osler, W. Gulstonian lectures on malignant endocarditis: lecture I. *Lancet* 1885; 3210:415–8.

2 Osler, W. Gulstonian lectures on malignant endocarditis: lecture II. *Lancet* 1885; 3211:459–64.

3 Osler, W. Gulstonian lectures on malignant endocarditis: lecture III. *Lancet* 1885; 3212:505–8.

4 Hoen B, Alla F, Selton-Suty C, *et al.* Changing profile of infective endocarditis: results of a 1 year survey in France. *JAMA* 2002; 288(1):75–81.

5 Cabell CH, Jollis JG, Peterson GE, *et al.* Changing patient characteristics and theeffect on mortality in endocarditis. *Arch Intern Med* 2002; 162(1):90–4.

6 Murdoch DR, Corey GR, Hoen B, *et al.*Clinical presentation, etiology, and outcome of infective endocarditis in the 21st century. 2009, *Arch Intern Med* 2002; 169(5):463–73.

7 ACCF/ASE/AHA/ASNC/HFSA/HRS/SCAI/SCCM/SCCT/SCMR   2011 Appropriate use criteria for echocardiography. *J Am Soc Echocardiogr* 2011; 24:229–67.

8 Li JS, Sexton DJ, Mick N, *et al.* Proposed modifications to the Duke criteria for the diagnosis of infective endocarditis. *Clin Infect Dis* 2000; 30(4):633–8.

9 Habib, G. Management of infective endocarditis. *Heart* 2006; 92:124–30.

10 Habib G, Derumeaux G, Avierinos JF, *et al.* Value and limitations of the Duke criteria for the diagnosis of infective endocarditis. *J Am Coll Cardiol* 1999;33:2023–9.

11 Erbel R, Rohmann S, Drexler M, *et al.* Improved diagnostic value of echocardiography in patients with infective endocarditis by transesophageal approach. *Eur Heart J* 1988; 9(1):43–53.

12 Shively BK, Gurule FT, Roldan CA, *et al.* Diagnostic value of transesophageal compared with transthoracic echocardiography in infective endocarditis. *J Am Coll Cardiol* 1991; 18:391–7.

13 Sochowski RA, Chan KL. Implication of negative resuls on monoplane transesophageal echocardiographic study in patients with suspected infective endocarditis. *J Am Coll Cardiol* 1993; 21:216–21.

14 Vieira ML, Grinberg M, Pomerantzeff PM, *et al.* Repeated echocardiographic examinations of patients with suspected infective endocarditis. *Heart* 2004; 90:1020–4.

15 Bonow RO, Carabello BA, Chatterjee K, *et al.* ACC/AHA 2006 Guidelines for the management of patients with valvular heart disease. *J Am Coll Cardiol* 2006; 48(3):e1–148.

16 Evangelista A, Gonzalez-Alujas MT. Echocardiography in infective endocarditis. *Heart* 2004; 90:614–617.

17 Oh JK. *The Echo Manual.* Philadelphia: Lippincott, Williams & Wilkins, 2006.

18 Roy P, Tajik AI, Giuliani ER, *et al.* Spectrum of echocardiographic findings in bacterial endocarditis. *Circulation* 1976; 53:474–82.

19 Bashore TM, Cabell C, Fowler V. Update on infective endocarditis. *Curr Probl Cardiol* 2006; 31:274–352.

20 Karalis DG, Bansal RC, Hauck AJ, *et al.* Transesophageal echocardiographic recognition of subaortic complications in aortic valve endocarditis.Clinical and surgical implications. *Circulation* 1992; 86:353–62.

21 Daniel WG, Mugge A, Martin RP, *et al.* Improvement in the diagnosis of abscesses associated with endocarditis by transesophageal echocardiography. *N Engl J Med* 1991; 324:795–800.

22 Habib G, Hoen B, Tornos P, *et al.* ESC Committee for Practice Guidelines. Guidelines for the prevention, diagnosis and treatment of infective endocarditis. *Eur Heart J* 2009; 30:2369–413.

23 Vilacosta I, San Roman JA, Sarria C, *et al.* Clinical, anatomic, and echocardiographic characteristics of the aneurysm of the mitral valve. *Am J Cardiol* 1999; 84:110–3.

24 Stout KK, Verrier ED. Acute valvular heart disease: changing concepts in disease managament. *Circulation* 2009; 119:3232–41.

25 De Castro S, d'Amati G, Cartoni D, *et al.* Valvular perforation in left-sided endocarditis: a prospective echocardiographic and clinical outcome. *Am Heart J* 1997; 134:656–64.

26 Mugge A, Daniel WG, Frank G, Lichtlen PR. Echocardiography in infective endocarditis: reassessment of the prognostic implications of vegetation size determined by transthoracic and the transesophageal approach. *J Am Coll Cardiol* 1989; 14:631–8.

27 DiSalvo G, Habib G, Pergola V, *et al*. Echocardiography predicts embolic events in infective endocarditis. *J Am Coll Cardiol* 2001; 37:1069–76.

28 DeCastro S, Magni G, Beni S, *et al*. Role of transthoracic and transesophageal echocardiography in predicting embolic events in patients with active infective endocarditis involving native cardiac valves. *Am J Cardiol* 1997; 80:1030–4.

29 Vongpatanasin W, Hillis LD, Lange RA. Prosthetic valve endocarditis. *N Engl J Med* 1996; 335:407–16.

30 Mahesh B, Angelini G, Caputo M, *et al*. *Ann Thorac Surg* 2005; 80:1151–8.

31 Habib G, Thuny F, Avierinos JF. Prosthetic valve endocarditis: current approach and therapeutic options. *Prog Cardiovasc Dis* 2008; 50:274–81.

32 Piper C, Korfer R, Horstkotte D. Prosthetic valve endocarditis. *Heart* 2001; 85:590–3.

33 Uslan DZ, Sohail MR, St Sauver JL, *et al*. Permanent pacemaker and implantable cardioverter defibrillator infection. *Arch Intern Med* 2007; 167:669–75.

34 Sohail MR, Uslan DZ, Khan AH,*et al*. Management and outcome of permanent pacemaker and implantable cardioverter-defibrillator infections. *J Am Coll Cardiol* 2007; 49:1851–9.

35 Vilacosta I, Sarria C, San Roman JA, *et al*. Usefulness of transesophageal echocardiography for diagnosis of infected transvenous permanent pacemakers. *Circulation* 1994; 89:2684–7.

36 Victor F, De Place C, Camus C, *et al*. Pacemaker lead infection: echocardiographic features, management and outcome. *Heart* 1999; 81:82–7.

Post-procedural complications

Vladimir Fridman

Cardiovascular Diseases, New York, NY, USA

Echocardiography is an extremely important test in the setting of post-procedural complications. It poses some very unique challenges to the echocardiographer, the most important of which is that the exact diagnosis is usually needed immediately.

Prior to performing a post-procedural echocardiogram, it is extremely important to know what procedure was performed. It is also absolutely necessary to know if the procedure was cardiac or noncardiac.

Noncardiac procedures

If the procedure was noncardiac, an echocardiogram is usually ordered for the following reasons:
- Hemodynamic instability/cardiac arrest
- Myocardial infarction
- Positive biomarkers post procedure
- Chest pain
- ECG changes
- Heart failure
- Failure to extubate patient
- Arrhythmia
  Most of these situations have been discussed in prior chapters.

Practical Manual of Echocardiography in the Urgent Setting, First Edition.
Edited by Vladimir Fridman and Mario J. Garcia.
© 2013 John Wiley & Sons, Ltd. Published 2013 by John Wiley & Sons, Ltd.

Cardiac procedures

If the procedure was cardiac, the echocardiogram needs to be tailored to look for specific post-procedural complications that could explain the clinical presentation.

Cardiac procedures include:

- Left and/or right heart cardiac catheterization.
- Percutaneous coronary interventions.
- Percutaneous valvular interventions.
- Electrophysiology studies/ablations.
- Pacemaker/ICD/cardiac arrhythmia device placement.
- Transvenous pacemaker placement.
- Pulmonary artery catheterization.
- Pericardiocentesis.
- Any cardiothoracic surgery:
  - valve repairs/replacement;
  - coronary artery bypass surgery;
  - cardiac transplantation;
  - lung biopsy/resection;
  - all other types of intrathoracic surgery.
- Cardiac biopsy.

If an echocardiogram is ordered after one of these cardiac procedures, it is important to know the exact reason for the order. Usually, there are specific diagnoses that must be ruled out post cardiac procedures. These are:

- Cardiac tamponade
  - This is the most important diagnosis to rule out in a post-cardiac procedure study.
  - ANY intracardiac procedure can cause bleeding into the pericardium and thus cardiac tamponade.
  - The presence of any size pericardial effusion should be worrisome.
  - Although pericardial effusions are common post cardiac surgery [1], if any hemodynamic instability is present, they are very important to diagnose and address medically.
  - Post cardiac surgery, the pericardial effusions can be small and be located in noncommon areas, such as behind the left atrium, but still be enough to cause tamponade physiology. This is especially true in the first 72 hours post cardiac surgery [2].
  - The presence of thrombus within the pericardium, especially post cardiac surgery, is able to cause tamponade physiology without pericardial fluid. In this case, the diagnosis should be suspected if there is evidence of increased central venous pressure (CVP), dilated IVC and/or SVC and a small right ventricle.

- If a pericardial effusion is noted, and the possibility of tamponade is raised, the patient's medical/surgical team should be immediately notified.
- Acute myocardial infarction
  - Very careful attention should be made to all the wall segments of the left ventricle (as described in prior chapters).
  - Any new wall motion abnormalities are concerning.
  - Overall systolic function should be carefully interrogated, and an ejection fraction should be carefully measured, and compared to any prior ejection fraction measurements.
  - Right ventricular function should also be noted, to make sure there is no acute RV infarction.
- Assessment of structure intervened on
  - This must be performed for every cardiac surgery case.
  - Very careful interrogation of the structure that was just intervened on should be undertaken
    - If a valve was repaired/replaced, multiple views, and all echocardiographic measurements, should be done to ensure the valve is working properly.
    - For cases where intracardiac shunts have been closed, careful Doppler interrogation of the area of the prior shunt should be done to exclude reopening of the shunt.
    - If aortic manipulation was done, multiple views of the aorta should be made to rule out any acute aortic pathology, as discussed in Chapter 8.
    - If an assist device was implanted, careful examination of the device, as described in prior chapters, should be undertaken.
- Acute valvular pathology
  - All valves should be carefully interrogated to rule out any acute regurgitant lesions.
  - Special attention should be made to all the parts of the valve apparatus, for each valve, so any new structural defect can be noticed.
  - Valves should also be assayed for presence of stenoses. Even though these are not acute conditions, they can cause periprocedural hemodynamic instability due to the effects of anesthesia/sedation on the flow through the stenotic lesions.
- Structural integrity
  - Careful interrogation of all the structures of the heart should be taken to make sure no acute ventricular septal defect (VSD)/wall rupture has taken place.
  - Color Doppler should be used in multiple views to make sure no intracardiac shunts, small or large, have formed post procedure.

- Right sided interrogation
  - Pulmonary embolus is a common complication of any procedure.
  - RV function and PA pressures should be recorded for all post-procedure echocardiograms.
  - Full pulmonary embolus evaluation has been described in prior chapters.

After a post-procedure echocardiogram is performed, the results should be quickly relayed to the medical team of the patient, especially if any positive findings are discovered. These echocardiograms are usually ordered in emergent situations, and a timely, accurate diagnosis via echocardiography can truly mean the difference between life and death.

References

1 Weitzman LB, Tinker WP, Kronzon I, *et al.* The incidence and natural history of pericardial effusion after cardiac surgery – an echocardiographic study. *Circulation* 1984; 69(3):506–11.
2 Price S, Prout J, Jaggar SI, *et al.* 'Tamponade' post cardiac surgery: terminology and echocardiography may both mislead. *Eur J Cardiothorac Surg* 2004; 26(6):1156–60.

"Quick echo in the emergency department": What the EM physician needs to know and do

Dimitry Bosoy[1] and Alexander Tsukerman[2]

[1]Department of Emergency Medicine, Maimonides Medical Center, Brooklyn, NY, USA

[2]Emergency Medical Associates, New York, NY, USA

CHAPTER 19

Focused cardiac ultrasonography (FOCUS) has been a bedside tool in the emergency department for years. Advances in ultrasound technology and the resultant creation of very small, portable, echocardiogram machines (hand carried ultrasound (HCU) devices) have made echocardiography a quick and easy bedside tool in the emergency department (Figure 19.1). FOCUS provides a great deal of anatomical and functional information. This modality is accurate, quick, noninvasive and readily available in most emergency departments. Physicians in the emergency department utilize FOCUS as an extension of the physical examination.

Goal of FOCUS

The goal of FOCUS in a symptomatic emergency department patient is to assess the following:
- Presence of pericardial effusion.
- Global cardiac systemic function.
- Identification of right ventricular diastolic collapse or strain and left ventricular enlargement.
- Determining intravascular volume.
- Guidance of pericardiocentesis and confirmation of transvenous pacing wire placement.

Practical Manual of Echocardiography in the Urgent Setting, First Edition.
Edited by Vladimir Fridman and Mario J. Garcia.
© 2013 John Wiley & Sons, Ltd. Published 2013 by John Wiley & Sons, Ltd.

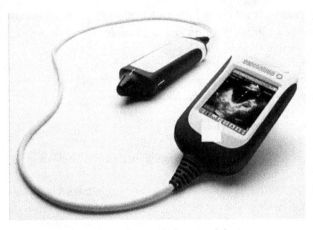

Figure 19.1 An example of a hand carried ultrasound device.

Pericardial effusions
- Are very easily identified by echocardiography.
- Detection of pericardial fluid requires knowledge of basic cardiac anatomy and identification of cardiac chambers.
- The pericardium is highly echogenic and is recognized anteriorly and posteriorly as a sonographic border of the cardiac image.
- Pericardial effusion appears as an anechoic space that separates the echogenic pericardium from the heart [1].
- Subcostal view is the most important view to evaluate for pericardial effusion in the acute setting.
- Most physicians use a 3.5-MHz transducer that can easily visualize all of the surrounding pericardium.
- The second view that is utilized in evaluating for pericardial effusion is a parasternal long axis view.
- Taking images in multiple windows can improve the sensitivity of the examination. Several echocardiographic signs of tamponade physiology have been characterized, but appreciation of such signs is sometimes difficult and requires experience.
- If pericardial effusion is visualized and clinical presentation is consistent with cardiac temponade then consultation with cardiology for a more comprehensive echocardiogram is warranted if time permits.
- The absence of pericardial fluids rules out the diagnosis of pericardial temponade.

Global cardiac systolic function
- Utilization of multiple windows, including subcostal, parasternal and apical, can differentiate patients with normal cardiac systolic function from depressed cardiac systolic function.

- The goal of FOCUS is to determine if a symptomatic patient has a depressed cardiac function and can benefit from specific pharmacologic intervention.
- A more detailed evaluation of cardiac function, such as segmental wall motion abnormalities, may require cardiology consultation and a comprehensive echocardiogram.

Right ventricular function
- Can easily be evaluated with FOCUS.
- In a patient with pulmonary embolism right ventricle may be dilated and dysfunctional.
- FOCUS can be easily used to identify hemodynamically significant pulmonary emboli by observing:
  - right ventricular dilatation, which is defined as greater than 1:1 RV/LV ratio;
  - decreased right ventricular systolic function or occasional visualization of free floating thrombus [2].
- Other pathology can cause right ventricular dilatation including:
  - pulmonary hypertension;
  - severe obstructive pulmonary disease;
  - severe obstructive sleep apnea;
  - right ventricular infarction.

The interpretation of FOCUS should be in the context of clinical presentation. A comprehensive echocardiogram should be performed for more detailed information when necessary.

Intravascular volume
- Accomplished by observing change in the diameter of the IVC.
- Done by viewing IVC below the diaphragm in a sagittal plane.
- IVC diameter varies with inspiration.
- The degree of inspiratory collapse of IVC can help determine the intravascular volume.
- Significant collapse of IVC signifies hypovolemic state.
- Putting together significant IVC collapse with hyperkinetic heart and normal right ventricular size can represent a hypovolemic state in a right clinical setting.

Clinical use of FOCUS

There are many clinical circumstances where FOCUS can play a role and affect clinical decision making in the emergency department:
- Cardiac trauma.
- Cardiac arrest or diagnosis of pulseless electrical activity (PEA).
- Undifferentiated hypotension/shock.

- Dyspnea/shortness of breath/pulmonary embolism.
- Chest pain and evaluating great vessels.
- Assessing for proper placement of pacemaker wires and guiding pericardiocentesis.

FAST examination

FOCUS has been incorporated into Advance Trauma Life Support and specifically into a Focused Assessment with Sonography for Trauma (FAST) examination.

- The FAST examination is used specifically to evaluate for pericardial effusions and can help determine which patient will require an emergent thoracotomy.
- Even a small effusion diagnosed by focused ultrasonography in a setting of trauma can lead to cardiac tamponade.
- Focused cardiac ultrasonography and FAST examination have been shown to improve outcomes by decreasing the time required to diagnose and treat cardiac injury.
- For more detailed evaluation of cardiac trauma, such as myocardial contusions, a comprehensive echocardiogram will be necessary.

Cardiac arrest

FOCUS is utilized more frequently now during cardiac arrest. The goal of focused cardiac ultrasonography during cardiac arrest is to:

- Establish cardiac standstill in a setting of electrical rhythm or PEA.
- Determine a cardiac cause for cardiac arrest.
- Assist with invasive procedures like pericardicentesis.

Most clinicians would agree that when echocardiography shows cardiac standstill it may be reasonable to consider termination of all resuscitative efforts, since return of spontaneous circulation is improbable.

Unexplained hypotension

- The goal is to immediately narrow the list of differential diagnosis of the shock state and initiate early and aggressive treatment.
- Simple assessment of global cardiac function and chamber size allows a clinician to assign a patient to one of four categories
  1. cardiogenic shock from severe left ventricular dysfunction;
  2. cardiac tamponade;
  3. massive pulmonary embolism;
  4. severe hypovolemia [3].

Evaluation of proximal IVC can contribute to formulating a diagnosis by establishing a right ventricular filling pressure. For example, hyperdynamic heart with significant inspiratory IVC collapse can signify a hypovolemic state and should initiate a search for hemorrhagic etiology of shock.

Dyspnea and massive pulmonary embolism

- Patients with a massive pulmonary embolism usually present in extremely unstable conditions and with impending cardiac arrest.
- Rapid diagnosis and treatment is vital to survival.
- The echocardiographic findings of massive pulmonary embolism include:
  - massive right ventricular dilatation;
  - right-sided heart failure with vigorous left ventricular contractility.

In addition, echocardiography can assist with excluding other causes that can mimic massive pulmonary embolism.

Aortic dissection and other great vessel pathology

- Occasionally, an aortic dissection can be detected on transthoracic echocardiography.
- A linear echogenic flap can be visualized across the aortic lumen.
- Most physicians utilize parasternal long and suprasternal long axis views to evaluate the aortic root.
- A transesophageal echocardiography (TEE) provides a much better resolution and visualization of aortic structures.
- If this is suspected, cardiology should be consulted and further imaging should be performed.

Overall, echocardiography has become an extremely helpful tool in the emergency department. With its portability and speed of image acquisition, echocardiography can be relied on in situations where an accurate clinical diagnosis must be established within minutes. For emergency department personnel, the knowledge of how to use this technology will become extremely important as it becomes the standard of care in the emergency department.

References

1 Plummer D. Primary applications of ultrasound: cardiac applications. In: Heller M, Jehle D *Ultrasound in Emergency Medicine*, 2nd edn. West Seneca, NY: Center Page Inc. Publishing, 1995: 126–34.
2 Labovitz AJ, Noble VE, Bierig M, *et al.* Focused cardiac ultrasound in the emergency setting: A consensus statement of the American Society of Echocardiography and American College of Emergency Physicians. *J Am Soc Echocardiogr* 2010; 23:1225–30.
3 Reardon RF, Joing SA. Cardiac. In: Ma OJ, Mateer J, Blaivas M. (eds), *Emergency Ultrasound*, 2nd edn. New York: McGraw-Hill Professional, 2007: 109–43.

Index

Illustrations are comprehensively referred to from the text. Therefore, significant material in illustrations (figures and tables) have only been given a page reference in the absence of their concomitant mention in the text referring to that illustration. Abbreviations used: FOCUS, focused cardiac ultrasonography; LA, left atrium; LV, left ventricle; RA, right atrium; RV; right ventricle; TEE, transesophageal echocardiography; TTE; transthoracic echocardiography.

Practical Manual of Echocardiography in the Urgent Setting, First Edition.
Edited by Vladimir Fridman and Mario J. Garcia.
© 2013 John Wiley & Sons, Ltd. Published 2013 by John Wiley & Sons, Ltd.